Patient Crisis
and Critical Thinking

Carol Whiteside, *MSN, PhD*

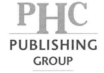

PUBLISHING
GROUP

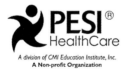

A division of CMI Education Institute, Inc.
A Non-profit Organization

EAU CLAIRE, WISCONSIN
2011

For information on this and other
PESI HealthCare products
please call 800-843-7763 or
visit our website at www.pesihealthcare.com

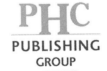

PUBLISHING
GROUP

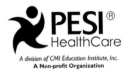

A division of CMI Education Institute, Inc.
A Non-profit Organization

Cover Design: Heidi Knower
Editor: Barbara Caffrey

Preface

It has long been my intention to expand my previous book *Subclinical Signs of Impending Doom* to include concepts of critical thinking and a model for integrating it into clinical practice. The main adage of critical thinking is that you cannot think critically about something that you know nothing about. Knowledge without action is wasted. The two – critical thinking and knowledge – must be combined for good patient outcomes, but getting there can be very difficult. I hope with this new, longer book (appropriately re-titled *Patient Crisis and Critical Thinking*) that both will be well served.

The first component of this book remains the knowledge section. New to this edition are added chapters regarding the concept of critical thinking along with a model for teaching critical thinking in the clinical setting. This model has been found to increase critical thinking in the people scoring toward the lower end of the bell-shaped curve before the model was introduced to them in a clinical trial.

We all want nurses to make the decisions that are best for their patients. But what is best for any patient changes as circumstances change. This is one of the hardest concepts to teach. Everything always depends on the context in which it appears. A low hematocrit on a post-partum mom and the same low number in a GI bleed patient will carry two different weights.

The critical thinking model takes this into account when it asks, "What *else* could be causing this to happen?" or, "What else would you like to know about this situation?" This model asks the nurse to go from "What happened?" to "Why did it happen?" The model is all about possibilities – what could the problem possibly be and what could have possibly caused it to happen? This is a big shift from task-oriented nursing to critical thinking (asking the question "Why?") because this model allows the nurse to look into the future for potential problems. Using the model gives both students and working nurses a framework for organizing their thoughts and coming to decisions.

I hope you find this book useful in your own practice and as a means of teaching critical thinking to your students. Just remember, the knowledge comes first, then the experience, and then, finally, the critical thinking. Omitting any one of these components will negate the whole.

Carol Whiteside, MSN, PhD
June 8, 2011

Introduction

Human physiology is like a choreographed ballet. It is gentle and it is fierce. It is logical and it is obedient. If everything performs as it should, there is health. If an event does not obey the rules, there is dysfunction and illness. All we have to do is figure out what the rules are. But the problem with the rules is that our understanding of them keeps changing as our knowledge of how the body works increases. Change is occurring faster today that at any other time in history and it shows no sign of slowing down. Nurses care for patients with higher acuity rates than ever before. What you are expected to know and do is through the roof! Your job is not one of crisis management, it is one of crisis prevention.

To prevent a crisis, you must be able to see it coming before it arrives. *Clinical* signs are the ones they taught us in nursing school: vital signs, lung sounds, neuro-vascular checks, etc. These signs are great for recognizing a problem because they occur *after* the body's compensatory mechanisms have failed to correct the problem.

What if we could see signs that compensation was taking place before the process failed? We can. It is these *subclinical* signs of impending doom that this book will depict – how to tell your patients are going bad before they keel over and die.

Everything – every thought, every movement, and every action in the body – has a physiologic, and therefore chemical, basis. The smallest living units in the body are its cells. It is the action and events occurring on a cellular level that spell wellness or illness in the human body. It is imperative that we know something about cellular metabolism in order to understand the compensatory mechanisms we want to observe.

Florence Nightingale said it is the physician's job to take the bullet out of the patient. It is the nurse's job to place that patient into the very best environment for healing to take place. She knew that you cannot heal your patients; patients heal themselves. Medical professionals bring bones together with all kinds of fancy screws and plates, but the patient must heal the break by himself.

What we nurses are equates to environmental engineers. We manipulate the environment and hope our patients have the wherewithal to heal themselves. The environment we manipulate contains things like inspired oxygen, giving drugs on time, making sure our patients have adequate nutrition, and keeping our patients in a safe place where they can heal.

Table of Contents

Chapter 1

The Cell

The Cell and the City

The first thing that I need you to do is to have what is called a "paradigm shift." By that, I mean that you need to stop thinking about things in the same way you always have and start thinking about them differently. The paradigm shift that you need to consider right now is this: stop thinking about your patients as macro individuals. Instead, start thinking about them as very large collections of microscopic cells. Then, remember that every single cell a human body is a living, breathing entity all by itself. When you die, you die one cell at a time. When you save someone's life, you do it one cell at a time. The more living individual cells there are in a patient's body, the more likely you are to have a living patient.

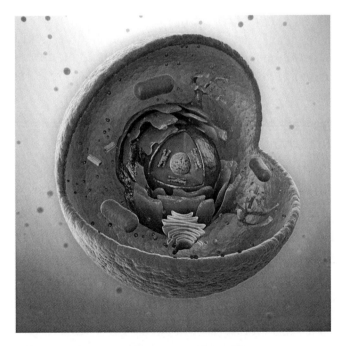

Figure 1-1. The Cell

All cells possess the same needs, wants, and dynamics as a city. Every cell in the body has to have and be able to do everything that a city has to have and be able to do.

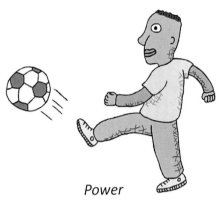

Power

Power in the City

A city must have a source of power. No power, no city. The more sources and quantity of power there are, the bigger the city gets to be. We use power to heat our homes, run farm machinery, manufacture and transport goods, maintain our health...countless things which could not occur without power. If we had no source of power, we would be back in the Stone Age at a time before the discovery of fire.

Power in the Cell

Inside the cell there must be a source of power. For the human body there is one source of power – Adenosinetriphosphate – or ATP. If you fire a neuron, you use ATP. If you contract a muscle, you use ATP. If you make a new red blood cell, you use ATP. It is the only source of energy in your body. It is made in the cell in the structure called the mitochondria. The number of mitochondria you find in a cell is directly proportional to the amount of energy that cell needs to produce. For example, hummingbird wings have ten times more mitochondria that the average bird wing muscle has. Do you see the analogy there? Which has more mitochondria: cardiac or skeletal muscle? Why? That's right: cardiac cells have more mitochondria because they must work continuously.

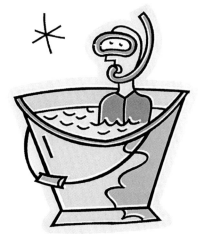

Water

Water in the City

A city must be near a source of water. No water, no city. The larger the source of water, the bigger the city can become. You do all kinds of things with water in the city; you drink it, you wash things in it, you cook with it, you float things on it for commerce, and you splash in it to cool off. Every city has a source of water and the city depends on the continued presence of water for its continued existence.

Water in the Cell

In the body there are several places for water to be: inside the cell (intracellular), outside the cell (extracellular), and in the vascular space (within the blood vessels). Maintaining the proper amount of fluid in these spaces is crucial for the life of the macro individual. So much so that if the volume (and thereby the pressure) is dropping off in the vascular space, the body will draw from the extracellular space to fill the vascular space back up. Then as the extracellular volume (and thereby the pressure) drops off you will draw fluid from the intracellular space to refill the extracellular space. Patients who are so severely dehydrated that they have sunken-in eyeballs have depleted all three spaces.

By the same token, if the volume (and thereby the pressure) increases in the vascular space, fluid is forced out into the extracellular space. This is the mechanism for ankle edema, ascites, pulmonary edema, etc.

As the extracellular volume increases, it will force fluid into the intracellular space. Having the right amount of fluid in the right spaces is crucial to the life of the macro individual due to the workings of the *micro* individual, or the cell.

Inside the cell, there are all kinds of little organelles and structures that make the cell work. If the cell is dehydrated, these things are all shrunken in on themselves, and they don't work right. If the cell is over hydrated, these structures get pulled apart, and again, they don't work right. The proper functioning of the cell requires proper fluid volumes in all spaces.

Your body is equipped with all kinds of sensors monitoring how things are going in your body. One set of these sensors are called *osmoreceptors*. They look at the *osmolality* – the concentration or dilution – of your blood. The osmoreceptors are tied directly into your thirst mechanism. If your blood is becoming concentrated, you *will* go get something to drink. Have you ever noticed how much patients *hate* being placed on fluid restrictions? Patients placed on fluid restriction have been known to drink from the toilet. Imagine how strong an urge would have to be for you to take a cup from the kitchen, go down the hall to the bathroom, scoop water out of the toilet, and drink it down.

That's how strong your thirst mechanism is. You will drink from the toilet before you will allow yourself to die of thirst. So if you put someone on a fluid restriction, you are asking them to go against what is probably his second-most basic drive. The body's most basic drive is take a breath, the second being to balance its fluids. Balancing fluids is essential to the functioning of the cells and therefore is essential to life.

If the thirst mechanism is so strong, why is it that elderly people are so often admitted to the hospital dehydrated? The answer is that if you live long enough, everything in your body will eventually fail you – including your thirst mechanism. With a younger person, no one needs to tell him to go take a drink of water when he's thirsty; the trick instead would be to hold him back! But the older someone gets, the less brisk his thirst mechanism becomes, which is why little old people don't always know when to take a drink of water.

When you are working with the elderly, you must frequently offer them something to drink. You must expect some of the patients to reply, "Oh, no thank you, dear. I'm not thirsty." As the nurse, you must tell your elderly patients to drink to maintain their health. Don't be afraid to say, "*Drink it!*"

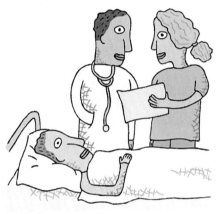

Food

Food in the City

It is easy to buy pineapples, wheat, or rice in the city, but chances are good that they are grown outside the city. That means there needs to be an intricate system of importing and exporting to get all the things you need into your city. Open lines of transportation and vehicles of some type are required. If the city's means of importation should break down, the city's vitality would be seriously curtailed – and it could possibly die.

Food in the Cell

The cell also needs food. Have you ever wondered what you do with the food you eat? Before you store it on your hips, there are three crucial things you do with it: you make energy from it , you repair your infrastructure, and you "make stuff" out of it.

Right now, your body is making epinephrine. It is making red blood cells. It is making all kinds of things from the food you eat. If you didn't eat it, inhale it, or absorb it through your skin (unless someone injected something into you), it isn't a part of your body.

When your body makes a new red blood cell, it lasts about 120 days. A neutrophil lasts only 24 hours, so every 24 hours you have to make new neutrophils as front-line defenders against infection. If your patient has an albumin of less than 1.5, they physiologically lack the building blocks (biological substrates) to make a scar. You must give people the building blocks to make things like an active immune system or a normal hemoglobin, and building blocks come from the food we eat.

Feeding our patients is not easy. Many patients challenge our ability to be creative, but you can't just *not* feed them. They can't heal themselves if you don't give them the building blocks with which to do it. Use your clinical dietician to find some way to get nutrients into the patient; if you can't, your patient could dehisce, be anemic, or become infected. Patients make scars, fresh red blood cells, and most importantly, active immune systems – everything they need – out of the food they eat.

Getting the biological substrates that have been eaten out to the cells requires an intact circulatory system. Have you ever had a patient with a non-healing ulcer on his foot who was sent away for an arteriogram? You may have been thinking, *"Why is he going for an arteriogram? What he needs is an antibiotic."* But if there isn't an intact circulatory system into the ulcer, there's no way to get the antibiotic down and into it. You must eat the biological substrates, but you must also have an intact circulatory system to get it out to where it needs to be used. If you can't improve the blood flow, amputations are often required.

Getting substances into and out of the cells is not an "everything-in, everything-out" proposition. There is a system of selectivity in the cells. If you want a substance to have an effect inside a cell, you must have a gate or receptor site for that substance. This makes good sense. You can't have every cell responding to every chemical floating in the bloodstream. For example, if you want Angiotensin II to have an effect, you must have an Angiotension II receptor site. Otherwise, it will just float on by in the circulatory system.

Receptor sites are very dynamic. If you block one of the receptors with a beta blocking agent (beta blockers block beta receptors on the cell membrane) the cell will respond to the lack of expected input by up-regulating the number of beta receptors on the cell membrane. This is because the cells in your body are aware of their environment; they know what is happening close to them and all throughout your body. The beta blocker dose must then be increased to block the new receptors. For this reason, patients must never abruptly stop taking beta blockers. They must be weaned off their beta blockers to allow the cells to down-regulate receptors on the cell membrane.

We have also learned that you up- and down-regulate these receptors from the cell membrane based on your circadian rhythms. The chemicals floating around in your bloodstream affect you differently at different parts of the day. (This is one reason why night shift is so physically and mentally difficult for most of us.)

One substance cells require more often than not is glucose. Cells use glucose to make energy. If your patient has a blood sugar of 450, his energy level is terrible. This is an indication that the glucose is not in the cell but is, instead, out in the bloodstream. We give the patient insulin to drive glucose back into the cell; it's a marvelous hormone that binds to the glucose in the circulatory system. On the cell membrane, there is a gate. Insulin holds the key to that gate. It binds to the glucose, opens the gate, brings the glucose into the cell, drops it off where the mitochondria can make ATP out of it and up goes your patient's energy level. A patient with a blood glucose of 450 and one with a blood glucose of 25 have the same pathetic energy level because glucose is not getting into their cells. Glucose must be inside the cells or it might as well not be there at all.

We Don't Know What We are Doing

We want the best for our patients. Unfortunately, we don't always know what we are doing. At any given moment in time, half of what we are doing is wrong. The only problem is that we don't know which half it is. What this means is that we have to stay current on the latest research and, in medicine, new research means things change constantly.

We do things because they look like a really good idea at the time, and then someone will come along and do a study disproving the effectiveness of the therapy and we stop doing it. For example, remember prophylactic lidocaine drips on rule-out MI patients? In the good old days, if a patient was a rule out, you bolused him and put him on a lidocaine drip. If he had more than five PVCs in a minute, two that looked different from each other, or two that touched each other, you bolused him again and turned the drip up, and up, and up. Then someone came along and did a study and discovered that the patients on lidocaine drips did worse that those without them. It turned out lidocaine is a myocardial depressant, so we stopped using lidocaine on patients with asymptomatic dysrythmias.

Or, remember aminophyline? If a patient wheezed once in the emergency room, he came to the floor on an aminophyline drip. Until someone came along and did a study that found that patients on aminophyline tended to have lethal dysrythmias brought on by the increase in their heart rate caused by the drug. So now, how many aminophyline drips do you have going on your floor? Almost none, with the only ones being used for the patients who can tolerate the increase in heart rate – like pediatric patients.

The term *diabetes* is yet another good example of how we don't always know what we are doing. When I got out of nursing school in the early 1970s I knew what a diabetic was. There were two kinds: adult and juvenile. But then some of the adults started getting juvenile diabetes, and some of the juveniles started getting the adult form. So we decided to call the two forms *insulin dependent* and *non-insulin dependent* diabetes.

But then, some of the non-insulin dependent diabetics became insulin dependent and then became non-insulin dependent again. So we gave them nice, non-descriptive terms: Type I and Type II diabetes.

But now we have another problem. What about the patients called *insulin resistant* or *glucose intolerant*? Are we looking at possibility of a *Type III* diabetes? Type I is a failure to produce insulin, Type II is a problem with the gate, Type III may become a problem with the key.

Worse yet, there is also a *Type 1.5*, or hybrid, diabetic. This is a Type II who has gone on to become totally insulin dependent, because we know that a percentage of Type IIs can become totally insulin dependent and – just like a Type I – they can also go into DKA. The most interesting thing about the Type I and the Type 1.5 is that their pancreases appear the same morphologically.

We all know about the rise of Type II diabetes in our society. Did you know the rate of Type I is also going up in similar numbers? That doesn't make any sense if they have two different causes.

All of that clearly indicates that nursing in particular, along with medicine as a whole, remains constantly in a state of flux. You must stay up on the latest research. We don't know anything for sure, except that we all were born and, eventually, we all will die.

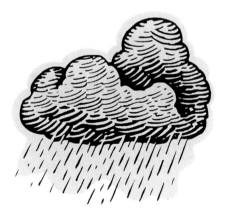

Storm Drainage System

Storm Drainage Systems in the City

From time to time it rains too much in the city, which is why cities have storm drainage systems to carry the water out of the city to the river, lake, ocean, or aquifer where it goes back into the ecosystem – in effect, a form of recycling. Without this protective device, cities would stay wet much longer and have more damage from flooding.

Storm Drainage System in the Cell

The body's storm drainage system called the *lymph* system. We constantly produce too much fluid around our cells, because the fluid is picked up by the lymph system, the debris filtered out in the lymph nodes, and the pristine fluid is dumped back into the central venous system and recycled. On a good day, this works very well for us.

There is, however, another fluid problem in the cell that requires a very specialized sump system. Ions flux in and out of the cells all the time for many different reasons. One ion that comes in a lot is Calcium. This wouldn't be a problem except that frequently when Ca++ comes in, it is holding the hand of its friend Na+. This also wouldn't be a problem, except that most Na+ ions have seven water molecules attached to them. If all this sodium and water were allowed to stay inside the cells they would swell up and burst.

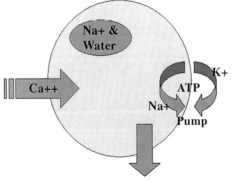

Na+ and water back out

Figure 1-2. Na+ K+ ATP Pump

To fix this problem, on the walls of every single cell in your body you have Na+ – K+ – ATP pumps to remove all that sodium and water. This is the largest use of energy in your body. As soon as your patient stops making ATP in sufficient amounts, every single cell in the body begins to swell up, and if left unchecked the cell will eventually burst. When one cell swells up and bursts it is called *lysis*. When many cells in one area sell up and lyse, it's called *necrosis* and, as you well know, when something becomes necrotic, it is never coming back again.

When you save someone's life, you do it one cell at a time. You die one call at a time and you save someone's life one cell at a time. The very first thing that you have to do to save someone's life is to keep those Na+ – K+ – ATP pumps running. The way you do that is by oxygenating and perfusing *at the same time*. You cannot do one at expense of the other. They must be simultaneous. As soon as oxygenation or perfusion is neglected, the cells begin to swell, become dysfunctional, and eventually undergo lysis, never to return again.

If a young, healthy patient is in shock, you may feel that if you can just get some fluids and drugs going, you should be able to save him. You may be surprised when this patient dies anyway. It all has to do with total number of cells left alive at the end of the untoward event and whether or not oxygenation and perfusion were maintained.

One night, a group of young men were driving around in a car with a gun. They were playing around with the gun when it discharged and blew apart one kid's femoral artery. At that point, all the kids in the car panicked. They were not supposed to be together, much less in a car with a gun, so they continued to drive around for awhile trying to decide what to do while the victim bled out. By the time they realized that they had a problem they couldn't deal with, they had stopped at a rest stop on the Interstate, which put them even further from help.

When the paramedics got there, they pulled the young man out of the car, started CPR, and got some lines and fluid into him. The paramedics said there was five inches of blood on the floor of the car. They brought the young man on into the ED, where they worked on him for about an hour and a half. Eventually they got some semblance of a heartbeat and blood pressure back. At that point, he was sent to surgery to have his femoral artery repaired. Since no one dies in surgery, he officially died in PACU. He went into Disseminated Intravascular Coagulopathy (DIC), used up all his clotting factors making microscopic clots, and bled to death (again). This young man had suffered so much cellular death before the paramedics even arrived that was truly nothing to get back. If you ever save a patient who marginally has just enough cells left to be alive, he is usually so severely damaged that you may wish you had never begun resuscitation.

To save someone's life, you must oxygenate and perfuse at the same time. Keep those Na+ – K+ – ATP pumps running. If the patient is breathing and oxygenating well, you don't have to do a thing. If not, step in immediately and breathe for him. If there is a good heart rate and blood pressure, nothing more is required from you. But if there isn't, step in immediately and get that heart rate and blood pressure adequate or the cells will begin to lyse. Remember that the more cells the patient has left alive, the more likely you are to have a living patient.

Another way to think about it is with regards to cardiopulmonary resuscitation (CPR). CPR teaches you ABC: Airway, Breathing (oxygenation) and Circulation (perfusion). Keep this in mind.

Whenever you enter into a patient care situation (remembering that every patient has his own special situation), you must know your therapeutic goal. If you don't know what your goal is, your therapy will be scattered. The primary goal of therapy should be to *always* oxygenate and perfuse at the same time. Everything else comes after that. This is so important that you might want to have this phrase, "Oxygenate and perfuse at the same time," tattooed onto your inner arm. That way, the next time a crisis hits and you think, "What do I do? What do I do?," you'd be more quickly reminded to oxygenate and perfuse at the same time.

This cannot be restated often enough: oxygenate and perfuse, at the same time. That's the primary goal. Everything else must come after that.

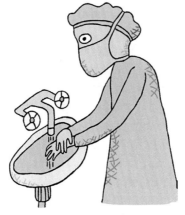

Sanitation

Sanitation in the City

Back in the 1800s Victorians didn't know what caused disease. Lister and Pasteur had just discovered the link to disease: microscopic organisms. John Snow had just determined that cholera was water-borne and came from one well in London. But as pedestrian as this seems to modern readers, at the time of these discoveries, this information was not met with universal acclaim; in fact, it caused a raging debate. Some people said, "Yes, I see the little beasties and they cause disease." Other people said, "You've got to be kidding. Disease is not spread by little beasties. It's spread by evil humors – bad smells."

Florence Nightingale was a member of the evil humor group. When she served in the Crimean War hospitals she had the floorboards, which had been soaked in human excrement, pulled up and replaced because they smelled bad. She had green scum washed off the ward walls because it smelled bad.

In those days, mattresses for sick soldiers were made of straw. Nurses would put a soldier on a straw mattress, then he would weep all sorts of nasty things on to it, then die on it. Seventy percent – 70% – of the soldiers who died in hospitals did not die of war wounds. Instead, they died of typhoid, cholera, typhus, and various other forms of dysentery. Now, imagine the mattress. While the dead soldier's body is sent to the cemetery with 8,000 of his fellow soldiers who also died in those hospitals, the next sick soldier was admitted and given the dead one's mattress and blanket.

Nightingale said that practice "smelled bad." So, under her care, every soldier got his own fresh mattress, his own freshly-washed blanket, and the nurses started doing something revolutionary – washing the patient's bed shirts. (It had never been done before.) Nightingale also pushed very hard for what she called "special diets for the sick." At this time, the rations for the well, healthy soldiers along with the ones dying in the hospitals was exactly the same – and many of the patients couldn't eat it. Nightingale changed this, which got nutrients into her patients. With her changes, she saw the death rate in her hospital go from 42% down to 2%.

Nightingale is well known for never ascribing to the germ theory of disease. She was very enamored over the science of hygiene. Think about it – most people back then had no idea what causes disease, which is why often, no effort was made to clean up excrement or dead animals. One of the doctors who served in the Crimean War said in a letter home to his family that the flies were so bad they got into his mouth when he was trying to eat. Nightingale and her nurses wrote home about chasing and killing the rats in the hospitals. They wrote that these rats were so big they sounded like men coming up the stairs. The nurses had also noticed that the patients placed nearest the bathrooms were the first to die, but they thought it was from the atrocious smells. Turns out the 4,000-bed hospital was on top of a plugged sewer system. Nightingale got that fixed also.

If there was no sanitation in your city, how long could it exist? Probably not too long. The sanitary problems of the 1700s and 1800s occurred during the Industrial Revolution when cities became crowded as people flooded into them looking for work. The sanitary habits of the farm proved inadequate for crowded city slums.

In the city, there are different kinds of waste being produced, requiring different kinds of waste removal. There's human excrement, grass clippings, recyclables, and hazardous waste from the hospitals, among other things. Each of these requires its own waste management program so as not to harm the city.

Sanitation in the Cells

The same system is in the body. There are different kinds of waste being produced and different kinds of waste removal systems available. The kidneys, lungs, GI tract, and skin get rid of waste for us. When you have a chemical reaction inside a cell, you sometimes produce a toxic by-product. If you have another chemical reaction, and right away change the toxin into something that is not toxic, we say you buffered it. That is your intracellular buffer system.

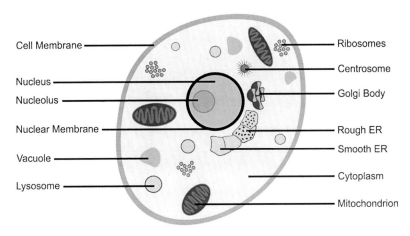

Figure 1-3. Lysosome

But sometimes you produce substances that are so toxic you can't buffer them. For these, you will need a specialized kind of waste removal system, and your body has one. It's called a *lysosome*. The lysosome is an organelle within the cell. The cell takes extremely toxic substances and encapsulates them because you can't have corrosive substances damaging the inner workings of the cell.

The cell moves these substances to the lysosome and dumps them in, because the lysosome contains extremely caustic enzymes that allow it to get rid of a nasty substance. That's the good part. The bad part is that those same extremely caustic enzymes contained within the lysosome are sitting right in the middle of the cell. If the lysosome's membrane should break down, the cell dies. And as this dead cell's membrane breaks down, the caustic enzymes come up against the membrane of the cell next door. The result is cascading cellular death, which is not good for a long and healthy life. Because of that, high up on your list of things to do should be to stabilize lysosomal membranes.

What causes lysosomal membranes to break down? First, if a cell swells up it can pull the lysosomal membranes apart. We will prevent that by oxygenating and perfusing at the same time to keep the sodium – potassium – ATP pumps running. The inflammatory process can also cause lysosomal membranes to break down, which in turn can cause the death of your patient. Prednisone is a drug that stabilizes lysosomal membranes in the face of inflammation so that, when you are done with your untoward event, you have more cells alive than you have dead. And that's a good thing. So we will oxygenate and perfuse at the same time to prevent cellular swelling and use prednisone in the face of inflammation.

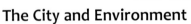

Environment

The City and Environment

Where you decide to put your city is dependent on the environment. If a city can respond and adapt to the environment, it thrives. If it can't, it dies. In cold environments, we have houses with roofs and heating systems. In hot environments, we have air conditioners. When Ann Brancroft and Liv Arnesen trekked across Antarctica, they hardly ran into anyone, because it was entirely too hard to respond and adapt to that environment for any human settlement to become established and thrive.

The Cell and Environment

The cells in your body also have an optimal environment determined by the pH. The pH in your body needs to be 7.35 to 7.45 – period. If the pH increases or decreases to an amount outside this range, every cell in the body becomes dysfunctional. Get far enough outside this range and the cells begin to die off. Your patient has got to have a normal pH or his individual cells will not function properly.

The human body does a great job responding and adapting to the environment. CO_2 retaining COPDers can become acidotic, but they retain bicarb and swing their pH back to normal. People in renal failure walk around with a BUN and Creatinine so high most of us couldn't stand up with it. People with chronic anemia walk around with hemaglobins so low that most of us couldn't sit on the side of the bed with it. If change happens slowly, the body does a wonderful job of responding and adapting. But if it happens quickly, the body may be in trouble. They say that what doesn't kill us makes us stronger, and that does appear to be true to a certain extent.

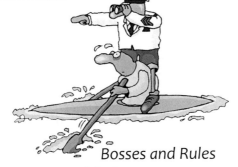

Bosses and Rules

The City, Bosses and Rules

Inside the city, you need a boss – someone to set the rules and keep law and order. Law and order is important, so the city can keep on with its day-to-day business and law-abiding people may leave their homes to go to nursing seminars. Would you have left home to go to a seminar if you thought there was a pretty good chance that when you came home your house would be ransacked and burned to the ground, and your children sold into slavery? Probably not. (Though it might depend on how your kids acted at breakfast that morning.) But, you are pretty sure that, when you get home at night, the kids will be right there with their hands stuck out and their mouths open. You don't have to camp out in the front yard with a shotgun, because we have rules that society follows. Usually.

The Cell, Bosses and Rules

Inside the cell, you need a boss. There is only one boss inside the cell and that is the DNA. The DNA makes any and all decisions. It is so important to the cell that it is encapsulated in its own nuclear membrane to protect it from the inner workings of the cytoplasm. If you should damage your DNA – and we do that from time to time – the cell takes a look at the DNA that comes before and after the break and tries to replicate the damaged part.

The rules for governing your body are strict. The rules are called *homeostasis* – the body's own equilibrium. Your body is an ultra right-wing fascist organization. There is no free thinking among the cells. Each cell will do the job it is born to do, never consider any other job, and work as hard as it can. When the cell can no longer put out at 100% effort, we kill it off and get a nice new cell to take its place.

We are happy because of this. We can't have pulmonary cells that decide they would like to be cardiac cells for a while. We can't have chemical messengers that decide that they will take a mental health day. We can't have cells that decide they want to spike their hair and pierce their nose, because when cells do that, they are called cancer cells.

Your body is making cancer cells right now. But instead of gathering them into little groups and rehabilitating them, your body is killing them off just as fast as it can. There is a cell in your immune system called a natural killer cell. This cell roams the body looking for cells that aren't with the program. It sidles up next to the malfunctioning cell, inserts a tube, injects a poison, pulls out the tube, and goes on its merry way looking for the next errant cell.

What did you make the natural cells out of? The only thing you making anything out of: the food you eat. How important is nutrition in preventing cancer? How much attention do we pay to it? How important is nutrition to cancer patients or any patient trying to fight off a disease? How much attention do we pay to it? We are getting better, but we still have a long way to go.

I have always said, "You are what you eat," but recently I heard an even better way to put this: "You are what your body does with the food you eat." That is most likely why there are different outcomes in different people.

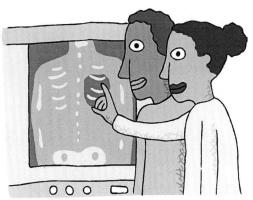

Infrastructure Repair

Infrastructure Repair in the City

As much as you hate it when they tear the roads up in your city, you would hate it a lot more if they A city repairs the roads, sewers, electrical systems, etc., on a near-constant basis. an ongoing project that consumes huge When funds are tight, infrastructure re things to get cut back. If this goes on lc into disrepair, becomes dangerous, a

Infrastructure Repair in the Cell

The same process is going on inside the cell and the body. We repair ourselves constantly. We repair our cell membranes, nuclear membranes, valve leaflets, gastric mucosa, skin, bones, and on and on. This repair is made with our reserve – what is left over after you are finished with beating your heart, digesting your food, breathing your lungs – left over nutrients and energy – are used to repair your infrastructure. Consider how quickly the human body decomposes. Up until the moment of death, the body was putting that much time and effort into making needed repairs. We may sag and we wrinkle, but we *don't* decompose.

The problem with some of our patients is that they don't have anything left over, so our job is to give them some reserve so they can make needed repairs. The component parts of reserve are: 1) biological substrates from food, 2) ATP as an energy source to work with and 3) an intact circulatory system to bring the good stuff and take away the bad stuff. This is the reserve we give our patients, then we sit back and hope our patients can heal themselves – because they are the only ones who can do it.

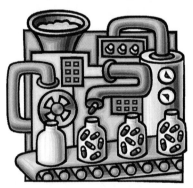

Manufacturing

Manufacturing in the City

Earlier, I had said that a city requires a vigorous import and ⁀rt system to get all it needs to function. That implies that there ⁀hing of value to pay for the imported goods. If the city sits ⁀ gold mine, all it needs to do is chip off little pieces of ⁀r things. But eventually the gold runs out; the city cuts down all the trees, kills off all the buffalo, and fishes out all the lakes and rivers – then what are they supposed to do? What's left for trade? At this point, many cities turn to manufacturing.

If you are going to manufacture something, the most efficient way to do it is inside a factory with an assembly line. Henry Ford taught us this. To make a car, the first thing you do is put down the wheels, then the engine, then the chassis, then the windows, and bingo! You've got a car. Because of this, it is going to be very important that things are in the right place on the assembly line. You can't have the windows at the beginning and the wheels at the end. Things must be in the proper order.

There must also be correct amounts of the various components for productivity. If you are running out of any one thing, say engines, you will be done making completed cars until you get more. So, someone has to be looking at the supplies on the assembly line. If engines are running low, they go back to their well-stocked warehouse, get more engines, put them in exactly the right spot on the assembly line, and go back and order more engines to restock the warehouse. It is a complex process designed to keep the assembly line humming along and productivity high.

Manufacturing in the Cells

This is exactly the same process used by your cells to make things. They use an assembly line called the *endoplasmic reticulum*. That endoplasmic reticulum has bumps along it called *ribosomes*. I use the analogy of a doll factory here to explain the relationship of these bumps to production of the completed substance. As the doll moves down the assembly line, the legs and arms are added to the torso. The head is attached and the dress placed on the doll to complete it. In smaller workshops, the face is painted and the hair added to the head. The head is then sent to the assembly line to be fixed to the completed doll. Another workshop makes the dress, or paints fingernails on the hands, etc. Those smaller workshops are the bumps on the endoplasmic reticulum. Amino acids, or whatever is needed, are assembled in the bumps and the component pieces are sent to the adjoining endoplasmic reticulum to be made into a completed product.

Let's say we have a cell that is going to make insulin. Insulin is a long chain amino acid. Where do the amino acids come from? From the food you eat. The smaller peptides and amino acid fragments come from the food you eat and are stored within the cell waiting to be used.

Cells makes insulin based on, among other things, your blood sugar. Which means the cell needs to know what your blood sugar is. You don't want it cranking out insulin if your blood sugar is low. Maintaining a normal blood sugar is actually a magnificent ballet between insulin, glucagon, and the somastatin produced in the GI tract. The following is only a small part of the show – the production of insulin.

On the cell wall, there is a sensor receiving information about your blood sugar. If the blood sugar is high, it causes the sensor to send a chemical messenger to the nucleus and the DNA to deliver the information. The DNA decides whether or not to make insulin. When the decision is made to make more insulin, the DNA does not leave the protection of the nuclear membrane. It sends its messenger, the RNA, out into the cytoplasm to the endoplasmic reticulum to deliver the news. So the messenger RNA goes out and says, "All right, guys, kick it up, we're going to make some insulin and here is the blueprint on how the DNA wants it done." The RNA's blueprint shows where to put which amino acids on the assembly line. Remember, some cells make more than one substance, so it has to decide what to turn on and off. Also, some hormones work by changing the contents of the blueprint which changes what the cell is going to make. The RNA's blueprint is the key to what the cell produces.

When you look at cells making things, remember there must always be a signal to turn the process on. We are pretty good at remembering that. Remember there must always be a signal to turn the process off. We are only fair at remembering that. But what we are awful at remembering is that you must get rid of whatever you made. How many gallons of epinephrine have you made in your lifetime? Where is it? How many swimming pools of cerebral spinal fluid did you generate last year? Where is it? How many trillion red blood cells have you made? Where are they? You must turn the process on, turn the process off, *and* get rid of whatever it is you made. There are three areas for disease to occur and three areas where drugs can work.

All right, so we are going to make insulin. The signal has come to turn the process on. Insulin is a long chain amino acid. Where did you get the amino acids from? Right, you ate them. They are transported to the cell via an intact circulatory system. The cell lines the amino acids up along the endoplasmic reticulum and a signal turns the process on. As the molecule of insulin comes down the assembly line, you add the first amino acid, then the second, then the third, etc., etc., until out the end comes a long chain amino acid called insulin.

When you look at a cell making insulin, it is not as simple as "make it and throw it into the blood stream." You need a reserve of insulin, don't you? (If you decide to have the chocolate mud pie after dinner, what happens to you if there is no reserve of insulin?) So, the cell is so sophisticated that when it makes the insulin, it looks at how things are in the bloodstream, the need in the reserve, and decides which way to go with this particular molecule of insulin. It's a very sophisticated process.

The Golgi apparatus is the storage mechanism within the cell. I like to think of it as the Amazon.com warehouse of the cell. Amazon takes your order, pulls the books and CDs from its shelves, drops them into a box with a big smile on the side, and mails them off to you. This is basically what the Golgi apparatus does. The substance is made, stored, packaged, and shipped based on orders from around the body.

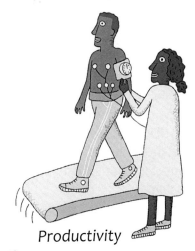

Productivity

Productivity in the City

The goal of manufacturing is productivity. To that end, you need healthy, motivated workers in sufficient numbers to get the job done. The reason you get days off from work is for your health. You are supposed to go home and rest so that you can repair your infrastructure and be more productive when you come back to work. (You do rest on your days off, don't you?)

Motivation is crucial to productivity. Have you ever worked with anyone who didn't share the group's common goal? Did that person harm the productivity of the group – perhaps so much so that you would like to open the ground, drop that person in, then cover him up and deny having seen him today? Productivity greatly increases if we are all working together to the same end.

Having the right number of healthy, motivated workers will ensure good productivity. Having too many workers strains resources. If you have too few workers, you can't get the job done. (For example, your hospital is always looking for the proper number of nurses. You always think it is one more and they always think it is one less.) Having the right number of healthy, motivated workers will ensure good productivity.

Productivity in the Cell

The cell is also concerned with productivity – getting done whatever it is supposed to be doing. A healthy cell is one with plenty of biological substrates, a repaired infrastructure, and lots of ATP available. As for motivation, among the cells there is only one, and that is to keep you alive. I said earlier that your body was an ultra right-wing fascist organization. It is also a perfect communist organization, because the idea behind communism is that everyone works at 100%, takes everything they make, puts it into a common pot, and takes back only what they need to be healthy and productive. But because human beings can often be greedy, selfish, and mean, it didn't work out at all.

But that is exactly how the human body works. As the nutrients, oxygen and other yummies float by in the bloodstream, the cells take only what they need. Your body doesn't have one cell stockpiling copper so that it looks cooler than the cell next door. They take only what they need and put back at 100% effort.

That holds true for most of the cells. There is one type of cell found in the human body that does *not* share the common goal, being an extremely greedy, selfish cell. When the yummies float by, these cells take everything they can reach. They will actually have blood vessels grow to them so they can get as much as they can from the available resources, all the while dumping their toxic waste back into the circulatory system. These, once again, are cancer cells. They care nothing about you – they care only about themselves, which is why they are so dangerous. But all the rest of the cells in your body are working together to try and keep you alive. You will see numerous compensatory mechanisms go into play to try and keep you alive before you are allowed to keel over and die.

It is the activation of some of these compensatory mechanisms that is the basis for the subclinical signs of impending doom. These signs are based in pathophysiology and are cellular in nature. Have you ever been blindsided by a catastrophic event with a patient at work, but when the crisis was over and you had time to think, you wondered, "Could I, should I, have seen it coming?" There is a saying in Radiology that states, "You only see what you know." What this means is that if you don't know something exists, you wouldn't be able to identify it if it was staring you right in the face. The rest of this book is to help you see and know what the signs are that the compensatory mechanisms have been activated. These signs are based in pathophysiology.

Key Components in Chapter 1

1. When you die you do it one cell at a time.
2. When you save someone's life you do it one cell at a time.
3. To keep cells from swelling up and lysing, you need to keep the sodium – potassium – ATP pumps running. You do this by oxygenating and perfusing at the same time – not one at the expense of the other.
4. Protect the integrity of lysosomal membranes by oxygenating and perfusing at the same time and using a steroid if there is an inflammatory process.
5. If you expect someone to heal, they need the biological substrates and ATP will be the energy source.

Chapter 2

Energy and Purpose

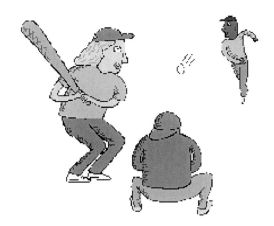

Adenosine Triphosphate

Let's revisit our friend adenosine triphosphate (ATP), the only energy source in the body. You make ATP via a process called oxidative phosphorylation. Oxidative phosphorylation is the most efficient way your body has to take the food that you eat and turn it into energy. It does it in the walls of the mitochondria via the Kreb's Cycle. (I do believe nurses were universally traumatized by the Kreb's Cycle in school. We do our very best to never think of it because it was such a disagreeable experience to see it appear on a test.)

Glucose + Oxygen = 37 ATP

What you should clearly remember about the dreaded Kreb's Cycle, however, is that if you have both oxygen and glucose and throw it into the cycle, ATP comes out the other end. With both glucose and oxygen present, you get 37 ATP every time you run the cycle and you obviously run it zillions of times to meet the body's needs.

Glucose without Oxygen = 3 ATP and Lactic Acid

Now, because your body wants to keep you alive, you can run the system without oxygen for a short time if you want to. But if you run it anaerobically, you only get three ATP each time. How is your patient's energy level as soon as they become hypoxic? How decreased the energy level becomes is directly proportional to how hypoxic they become.

Not only does the patient's energy level decrease, but they also begin to crank out lactic acid. The problem with lactic acid is that is upsets the body's pH which is the environment for all the cells. Every cell in the body becomes dysfunctional when the pH changes, and if it goes on long enough, the cells will start to die. The more dead cells you have, the more likely you are to have a dead patient.

Making ATP anaerobically is a short-term compensatory mechanism. You cannot live a long and healthy life if you are anaerobic. You need to find out what is wrong (is it a problem with ventilation, perfusion, or both?) and fix it before you end up with a dead patient.

$$Glucose + Oxygen = 37\ ATP$$

We have determined the lactic acid is produced by anaerobic metabolism. If you could then measure the amount of lactic acid in a patient's body, would you be able to extrapolate how much anaerobic metabolism is going on? Sure you can. Measuring lactate levels tells us the amount of anaerobic metabolism going on in the body; this is used to determine the severity of the problem in both septic and trauma patients.

Keeping the Heart Beating

If asked which organ is the most important in the human body, many people will say "the brain," because that is where the essence of the human being resides. (The ancient Greeks thought it resided in the liver). I don't know where the human spirit is located, but if you have ever had a brain-dead patient, you know that the rest of their body works just fine, thank you. But if you have had a heart-dead patient, you know that the rest of the body will only continue to work for a minute or two. When I ask what the most important organ in the body is, I'm really asking which organ kills you first.

When you die, one hundred percent of the time – 100% – you die from a lethal dysrythmia. You don't die from hypoxia, you die from the lethal dysrythmia caused by the hypoxia. You don't die from renal failure, you die from the lethal dysrythmia caused by the renal failure. When you go, one hundred percent of the time, you go from a lethal dysrythmia. So, let's take a look at what you have to do to keep someone's heart beating.

The EKG tracing you see running across the screen does not signify squeeze in the heart. It is an *electrical request* for a squeeze. It asks, *"Please squeeze now if you don't mind."* Most of the time the heart says, *"Sure, I don't mind,"* and squeezes. But not always. It is possible to get a beautiful electrical request for squeeze and therefore a beautiful EKG, but still have no squeeze. This is called pulseless electrical activity (PEA). But most of the time when asked, the heart agreeably contracts.

I said it was an *electrical request* for a squeeze, which means you generate electricity in your body – enough to run a hundred watt light bulb, I've been told. How do you do that? Here are your three possible answers. The first is, "I have a battery pack, but never told anyone." The second is, "I plug in at night but have never told anyone," while the third, and correct answer is, "I shift ions across a semi-permeable membrane." Where did you get the ions from? You ate them. Where do you get potassium from? Strawberries, oranges, bananas. You eat the ions and hope they don't leave your body before you need to use them.

The Four Requirements for a Happy Heartbeat

If you placed an electrode inside a myocardial cell and watched the electricity course through it, this is what you would see on your oscilloscope. This is your action potential.

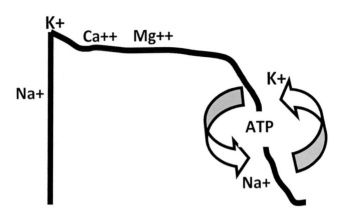

Figure 2-1. Action Potential

The sharp upstroke is caused by Na+ rushing into the cell: the peak is a Na+ overshoot mediated by potassium (K): the plateau is where Ca++ sustains the squeeze; and Mg++ is used for membrane stability by moderating the flow of potassium and sodium in and out of the cell. This sequence causes depolarization and the ensuing electrical request for the heart to contract.

Now that we have depolarized, we must repolarize and to do that we need energy. The only energy we have is ATP and we will run another Na+ – K+ – ATP pump to shove those ions back across the electrical gradient on the cell membrane and get ready for the next heartbeat. The Na+ – K+ – ATP pumps appear all over the body doing all kinds of different things, but what they are doing here is repolarizing the cell membrane's electrical gradient and getting ready for the next heartbeat. Remember, if you can't repolarize the last one, there will not be a next one.

There are four things that must be perfect for the action potential to work and for the human heart to beat.

1. You must have a normal pH (the environment for cell function),
2. All the electrolytes must be balanced to generate the action potential,
3. There must be oxygen, and
4. glucose inside the myocardial cell to make ATP to repolarize the cell and get ready for the next beat.

5. One hundred percent of the time when you die, you die from a lethal dysrythmia caused by an imbalance in one or more of the above requirements for a happy heartbeat. Take any disease process you can think of, work your way down to the moment of death, and you will find one or more of the four requirements out of alignment.

All the disease processes simply become conduits into a malfunctioning of the action potential's pH, electrolytes, glucose and oxygen. The end goal of oxygenating and perfusing (and the entire ACLS protocol) is so the patient will have a normal pH, balanced electrolytes, and oxygen and glucose inside the cell so that the patient can repolarize his action potential and get ready for the next heartbeat.

Digitalis

Earlier, I had said that Ca^{++} sustained the squeeze in the myocardial cell. If I wanted to invent a drug that increased myocardial contractility, do you suppose that having more Ca^{++} in the cell would do so? Of course it would, but there is a problem with the Ca^{++}. Remember, it was bound to the Na+ and water? To increase myocardial contractility, you want more Ca^{++} to stay behind in the cell, but you don't want the Na+ and water stay behind. That would cause the cell to swell up and burst. What you need is a drug that poisons the $Na^+ - K^+ - ATP$ pump on the cell wall so that the Na+ and water is pumped out but more Ca^{++} is left behind. This drug is called digitalis. Because of its interaction with the $Na^+ - K^+ - ATP$ pump, there are four things that must be absolutely perfect for a person taking digitalis:

1. You must have a normal pH (the environment for cell function),
2. All the electrolytes must be balanced to generate the action potential,
3. There must be oxygen, and
4. glucose inside the myocardial cell to make ATP to repolarize the cell and get ready for the next beat

If a patient has trouble with digitalis, it usually signals an electrolyte imbalance, but digitalis does not affect electrolytes.

What happened to the patient's electrolytes?

Remember in nursing school when you took a test? You might look at a test question and think, *"It depends."* You may have gone to the teacher and said, *"The answer to this question depends."* And she might have replied, *"You're reading too much into the question."* And you might have reiterated, *"But it depends!"* By this point, your instructor probably would've told you to knock it off, so you'd have gone back to your seat and made a guess. Well, nothing in nursing/medicine is linear. *"It depends"* is always the right answer.

When considering a situation you must consider all variables – other co-morbid factors, other drugs on board, other insults to the system that may be occurring, the patient's kidneys, his breathing, his nutritional status, and on and on. There are so many things that need to be considered. When trying to determine why a patient is having difficulty with digitalis, consider that it is usually the electrolytes that are off. Though digitalis didn't affect the electrolytes, the Lasix you gave him *with* the digitalis did. Or it could be his newfound renal insufficiency.

Patients who are CO_2 retaining COPDers will retain CO_2 and make themselves acidotic. People taking potassium-sparing diuretics can become alkalytic. Based on the four requirements for a happy heartbeat and the addition of digitalis, it seems to m, that you should never give digitalis to anyone who is a CO_2 retaining COPDer, anyone on Lasix, anyone who could ever become hypoxic, or anyone who was diabetic. But these are the patients who are most likely to get digitalis! Digitalis is an excellent drug, but requires a delicate balance in the patient and a vigilant nurse. If you have a patient with an imbalance in their pH, electrolytes, glucose or oxygen and they have digitalis on board, they are at high risk for a lethal dysrythmia and death. You must get it fixed!

Purposes of the Organ Systems

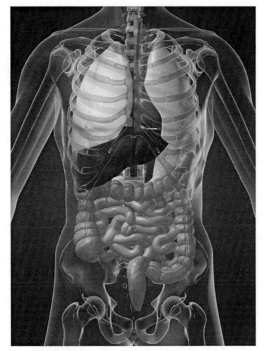

Figure 2-2. Organ Systems

In school, I studied the functioning and the A&P of the organ systems, but I don't remember ever looking at the purpose of those organs. So let's do that now.

GI System

What is the purpose of the GI system? It takes food from outside the body, breaks it into little, bitsy, tiny pieces (those biological substrates) and puts them where? Into the circulatory system. Where do they go from the circulatory system? Off to the cells. And what was it the cells did with the food you ate? Before you stored it on your hips, you made energy, made stuff, and repaired your infrastructure.

Respiratory System

What is the purpose of your respiratory system? It brings in air from outside the body, extracts the oxygen, and puts the oxygen where? Into the circulatory system. And from the circulatory system where does it go? To the cells. What did the cells do with that oxygen? They made ATP out of it. There are chemical reactions in the cells that require oxygen be present for them to occur (catalyst), but the vast majority of the oxygen you breathe in is used to make ATP.

Why will a patient who has stopped breathing die? Because there is no O2 for ATP to repolarize her action potential. If you can't repolarize your action potential and get ready for the next heartbeat to come along, there will be no next heartbeat – instead, you will have a lethal dysrythmia and die. The very first ATP that you need to make is that required to repolarize the last action potential. Everything else comes after that. So if your patient quits breathing, or isn't oxygenating well, you must jump in immediately and get them breathing again or sustain respiration for them before the lethal dysrythmia occurs.

Cardiovascular System

What is the purpose of the cardiovascular system? It is a transport media. That is all that it is. It brings the good stuff to the cells and takes the bad stuff away. What is the purpose of the heart? It is the pump that moves the transportation system. If the heart stops beating, good stuff stops coming to the cells, bad stuff stops going away, and very soon you will have dead cells. The more dead cells you get, the more likely you are to get a dead human being.

Renal System

What is the purpose of the renal system? What is it there for? One purpose is to rid the body of waste. One of those waste products is BUN – blood urea nitrogen. Where did it come from? It is an end product of protein metabolism in the individual cells. When you ask where something comes from in the body, the answer is always from the cells. You can say it comes from the tissues or from the organs, but guess what? They are made of cells. Remember those kidneys are also responsible for balancing your pH, electrolytes, and fluids – three things that can make you real dead real quick.

Musculo-skeletal System

What is the purpose of the musculo-skeletal system? What advantage do we have in being upright mobile creatures compared to if we were lying on the floor? What do we get because we can walk around? Our only energy source in the human body is ATP, made of oxygen and glucose. If we are hungry, we can go get something to eat. The amoeba has to wait for it to float by. It doesn't float by, the amoeba starves.

When we go get something to eat, we frequently go get something to drink. We can manipulate and manage our own body's fluid balance, which is crucial. But the amoeba is totally at the mercy of the fluid around it. If the pond dries up, the amoeba dries up, but we upright mobile creatures can attempt to control our own fluid balance. If we are thirsty we can get into the pool, swim down to the shallow end where there is a bar with palm fronds hanging down, and get something to drink to go with those fish tacos we just ordered.

If we can move toward good things, can we move away from bad things? Of course we can. If I hear the train coming; I will get off the train tracks. I will move out of the sun into the pool and order an iced tea from the cute bartender in the in-pool bar before I die of heatstroke. This is a nice manipulation of events and environment.

Because I am an upright creature, along with my backache I get the ability to see farther and hear better. I can put some of my sensory organs on a stalk and I can rotate them. In this way, you can hear, see, and smell more efficiently than if you were lying on the floor all the time. Being upright creatures gives us advance warning of good and bad things coming our way.

Nervous System

We have a fabulous nervous system – particularly when we are young. In later life it can, at times, leave something to be desired. It is believed that only human beings can predict the future. Can we really predict the future? You bet we can and we don't even need a crystal ball. If you decide to feed your two year old Brussel sprouts, do you know what will happen? If your fifteen year old daughter calls up and says she is spending the night with her boyfriend, do you know what will happen? If you get on *that* freeway at *that* time of day in *that* city, you know *exactly* what is going to happen.

Because we can predict the future, it can save us a lot of grief. Other animals can have a negative experience and learn to avoid the circumstances, but humans can look at a situation and say, "That doesn't look like a good idea to me!" and never have the negative experience. What a wonderful technique for preservation of the species.

Earlier I said that you had all kinds of sensors in your body looking at how things were going. What is looking at the input from those sensors and making adjustments? It is the part of the nervous system that you hated most in nursing school. You may have blanked it out of your conscious memory. It is our marvelous, amazing, *autonomic* nervous system.

We have a wonderful system that cranks us up in a time of stress and then brings us right back down when the stress is gone – the *sympathetic* and *parasympathetic* nervous systems. Why is it that we need to be cranked back down at all? Why can't you just stay sympathetically stimulated? Because you would look like a meth addict. You can't eat enough to generate the energy, repair your infrastructure, and make the stuff required to go full bore like that. So our system cranks us up in a time of stress and brings us right back down when the stress is gone.

Our bodies inside have changed very little since the caveman days. Outside, the environment has changed drastically, but inside we are pretty much the same as we have always been.

Imagine that you are living in the Stone Age. It is night time and you are outside warming your hands at the fire. You have your new cave skins on and you look very sharp tonight. All of a sudden, you hear a twig snap behind you, and you whirl around. Would it be advantageous to increase the blood flow up into your brain at this time? Why? What are you going to do with more blood in your brain? Think faster? How does more blood in your brain help you do that? You need oxygen? Oxygen for what? ATP! If you want to fire your neurons faster and heighten your senses, you need more ATP!

To get more oxygen, you breathe faster and deeper, your bronchioles get bigger, and dilating the blood vessels into the brain and increasing myocardial contractility and heart rate kicks up the transport system.

So you have your transport mechanism in high gear, and you've thrown in lots of oxygen, but ATP is oxygen plus glucose. So we'd better stop and get a sweet roll. No? Where are you going to get the glucose from? You get the glucose from your stores.

Just what stores are you thinking of? You had better not be thinking of your body fat. Your body guards its fat stores carefully because they are a survival mechanism. That fat is there for the great trek across the Sahara during the famine that is never going to come. Should you be so irresponsible as to lose some of your fat, your body will help you find it again and give you some extra in case you choose to act irresponsibly again. Your fat is your body's last choice when going after energy stores.

The first place you have stores are in the muscle cells themselves. You have three minutes of oxyhemoglobin that will get you up and get you going. In your liver you store glycogen – it can be thrown out into the circulation and be used by the cells to make ATP. But where next?

One hundred percent of the time, when you've crawled out of bed in the morning you have always been alive, haven't you? It is not unusual for you to not eat for hours before going to bed and not unusual for you to not eat for hours after you get up in the morning. What did you run your body on all night long while you weren't eating? Your body used the stores contained in the muscle cells themselves. Your body tears down the muscle cells into their little amino acid parts, releases them back into the bloodstream, and sends them off to the liver. The liver makes new sugar out of it with a process called *gluconeogenesis*. All night long you run on gluconeogenesis.

The next morning you get up, eat some amino acids for breakfast, and put them right back into your muscle cells. It is a continuous up and down replication process that works beautifully until you make someone NPO. (An abbreviation for the Latin term *nil per os*, meaning "nothing by mouth.") If you make someone NPO, his body goes immediately after his muscle cells. Remember that the heart and diaphragm are two large muscles you don't really want broken down for their stores. This is one reason why nutrition is so important.

When you make someone NPO, consider the whole history and the whole patient. I admitted a patient the other day who had ruptured a diverticulum. If you rupture something in your GI tract, the first thing you get is NPO. This lady was as big around as she was tall, so you would think she must have wonderful nutritional stores. (No, there is no correlation between the two.) I looked back in this lady's H&P and I see that six months ago, she had a hemicolectomy for colon cancer. Then she had radiation therapy to her gut and her body had never healed her primary surgical wound – she had a woundvac in it. Now what do you think about this patient's nutritional status? If you are going to make someone NPO, always say to yourself, "Does this person have the muscle mass to tolerate NPO?" And if the answer is, "No," use your clinical dietician to help you figure ways to get nutrients into this patient. Remember you make scars, red blood cells, and active immune systems out of the food you eat.

Let's go back to our sympathetically stimulated cave person. When you are sympathetically stimulated, do you digest your food? No, this non-essential function slows down. Are sympathetically stimulated people interested in sex? They shouldn't be. They need to be paying attention to their environment!

You hear a noise, turn around and look, and you see your friend behind you. You can't stay sympathetically stimulated – you need to be parasympatheticaly stimulated. Your heart rate goes down. Your bronchioles get smaller. Do you digest your food? Yes. Are you interested in sex? Perhaps, depending on who it is behind you.

The sympathetic system is "fight or flight," while the parasympathetic system is "feed and breed." We were designed to be much more parasympathetically stimulated than sympathetically stimulated. In our world, we tend to be too sympathetically stimulated and we have all kinds of health problems because of it. A lot of those problems are centered in the gut because the gut runs on parasympathetic stimulation. You were designed for a tropical island, not a hospital.

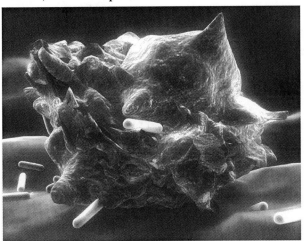

Figure 2-3. Macrophage

This is a type of macrophage. Did you make it out of the food you eat? Does it use ATP as an energy source? You bet. How well does it work when the body is hypoxic? Not so well. How does it work when the blood sugar is out of adjustment? Not so well. The problem with diabetics and infection is not that they don't have the macrophages – they usually do. The problem is that the macrophages are sluggish because they don't uptake the glucose in the blood the way they should to make ATP and run an active immune system. Diabetics are very prone to infections, especially when they are stressed. A correlation exists between blood sugar and complications. The closer the blood glucose comes to normal, the more complications just fall away.

If you want to get your patient back into a state of wellness, two things that you can do to speed them in that direction are to make sure they never become hypoxic (and if they do, get them out of it immediately), and keep tight control of the blood sugar. We are beginning to see patients on the hospital wards with insulin drips, lantus insulin, and coverage after meals as therapy because having a normal blood sugar is key to macrophage functioning and wound healing. Sliding scale coverage is nice, but having a continuous normal blood sugar is even nicer.

Key Components in Chapter 2

Oxygen plus glucose is how the body makes ATP using the Krebs cycle run in the walls of the mitochondria. O2 + glucose = 37 ATP

1. You can run the system without oxygen (anaerobically) but you only get 3 ATP and begin poisoning the system with lactic acid. Measuring lactate levels can tell you how much anaerobic metabolism is going on.
2. The heart beats in response to an electrical request for squeeze – it is seen as the PQRS on the EKG.
3. The four requirements for repolarizing the heart and getting ready for the next heartbeat to come down the conduction system are
   i. Normal ph
   ii. Balanced electrolytes
   iii. Glucose and
   iv. Oxygen inside the cell being used to make ATP
4. The organ systems are there to keep the individual cells alive and productive.
5. To maximize your patients' macrophages, make sure they are not hypoxic and have normal blood glucose.

Chapter 3

Oxygen Delivery to the Cells

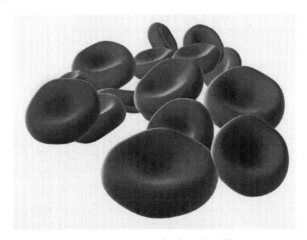

Figure 3-1. Red Blood Cells

These are red blood cells. These are what we use to deliver oxygen to our cells so they can use it to make ATP and/or be catalysts for other chemical reactions. The average red blood cell is one-tenth the size of the average cell so they can maneuver through the microvasculature serving the cells. The edges are smooth so they won't get stuck in narrow places, which is what causes ischemia and infarctions. Red blood cells also have a dip in the middle that increases the surface area for the binding of hemoglobin to the oxygen molecule. (It would be possible to get the same increase in surface area if the red cell bulged outward, but if that happened, you would have little bee-bees, which would not be capable of fitting into the same tight spaces the flexible red cell can.) That RBC can literally fold in half in a tight space and spring back to normal when the space is larger. They are slick, flexible, and fantastic. This is what we use to deliver oxygen to the cells.

Oxygen Transport to the Cells

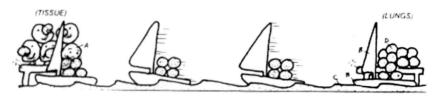

Figure 3-2. Normal O2 Transport

The illustration above goes from the right to the left, not left to right as do the words on this page. The component parts of delivering oxygen to the tissues are: the dock represents the lungs, the Os the oxygen molecules, the sailboats are the red blood cells, and the wind in the sails is the blood pressure. If you have functioning lungs, available oxygen, sufficient red blood cells to hold the oxygen, and enough blood pressure to carry it to the target, oxygen is delivered to the tissues.

But now, you get sick. Hypoxia is not a disease, but rather a symptom of something else going wrong. There are four types of hypoxia.

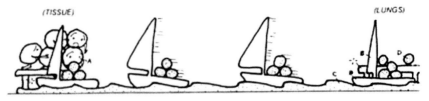

Figure 3-3. Hypoxic Hypoxia Transport

In a *hypoxic hypoxia*, insufficient oxygen has been delivered to the dock (pneumonia is an example), insufficient oxygen is loaded onto the red blood cells, and insufficient oxygen is delivered to the tissues. This irritates the heck out of those cells, they go anaerobic, stop working as well as they should, and begin pumping out lactic acid and poisoning the environment for all the cells. Not good. The treatment for this patient is oxygen. Intubate, trach, heliOx, *whatever – you* must get oxygen into the patient or he is going to die of a lethal dysrythmia caused by an inability to repolarize his action potential.

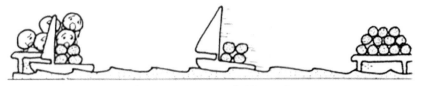

Figure 3-4. Anemic Hypoxia

In an *anemic hypoxia* the problem is that there are insufficient red blood cells to carry the oxygen to the cells. The cells could care less why the oxygen didn't arrive; it's just not there! The result is the same on the cellular level as hypoxic hypoxia: the cells get irritated, stop functioning properly, and crank out lactic acid.

What is your treatment for an anemic hypoxia? Add some red blood cells to the mixture, right? Maybe, maybe not. Nothing has changed more in my nursing career than who does or who doesn't get a blood transfusion. When I first got out of school, if a patient had a Hematocrit of less than 32 they got a transfusion. Not anymore. We had that little problem in the blood supply called the AIDS epidemic and it made us stop and look at the way we gave people blood.

A healthy teenager who suffered a trauma was sent home with an H&H of 15/5. Should this patient have been transfused before he was discharge? Consider that this teenager's bone marrow is in pristine condition. If you want him to make red blood cells, you feed him, and he will make them just as fast as he can. He will be tired and run down for a while, but he won't wake up with AIDS, hepatitis, or whatever else we might be passing around in the blood supply that we don't know about. When I got out of school we had hepatitis A, B, and non-A/non-B. We are now up to H in the hepatitis "family." Hepatitis C is not a new disease. It was always there; we just didn't know what was causing all that liver failure and liver cancer. We now know it was hepatitis C and we were passing it around in the blood supply.

Not giving someone a unit of blood is a really swell idea – if you can get away with it. Whether or not you can get away with it depends on four factors.

1. Who is the patient? What are his reserves? Did he have a lot of co-morbid factors going into the event or was he strong and healthy?
2. What is the nature of the event? Is it over or is it continuing? Was it severe or mild?
3. How much time do you have? If there is time, allow the patients to make their own new blood cells. No time? Transfuse immediately!
4. Is the patient symptomatic? If the patient is symptomatic, the other factors don't matter. Transfuse now if it is a viable option.

So, a decision to transfuse is dependent on multiple factors. There is no set number at which you do anything. A patient in cardiac arrest was admitted to the ER. His hematocrit was 32. For a patient who has just had a cardiac arrest, a hematocrit of 32 is entirely too low. He was promptly given two units of packed red blood cells. He needs oxygen carrying capacity.

Another patient was a twelve-year-old girl involved in a sled vs. MVA trauma. She had a liver laceration and was actively bleeding. We started pouring blood products into this young patient. The lab values came back and she had a hematocrit of 36. Should we have stopped the transfusions? No, because she was still actively bleeding. The event was not over.

I asked an OB nurse one day what was the lowest hematocrit she would allow a new mother to go home with. "Oh, I don't know," she said, "Ten, eleven, twelve. Somewhere around there." But, think about it. Here's a well, healthy individual (if she's not, it changes everything), the event is over, and she has the rest of her life to make red blood cells. You don't want to transfuse a healthy, young person if you don't have to because giving someone a transfusion can open up a Pandora's Box of complications.

But my best guess is that you don't work with a lot of healthy, young patients with good reserves. Your average patient is probably an elderly, chronically ill person, so you would be more likely to transfuse these patients sooner. It always depends on the patient, circumstances, time, and whether or not the patient is symptomatic.

New studies regarding the outcomes of patients in the ICU who were given transfusions versus those who were not have shown that the non-transfused group actually did better. Researchers are not sure why. More studies are ongoing.

If you want to know if a patient is making new red blood cells, take a look at the retic count. A reticulocyte is a brand new baby red blood cell. If the patient is reticing, you may be less likely to transfuse. We also have erythropoietin these days, which can stimulate someone's hematological stem cells to turn themselves into red blood cells. If a patient is getting erythropoietin or Neupogen, nutrition is crucial. You have to give the patient the biological substrates to make the red cells or they simply can't do it.

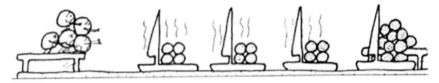

Figure 3-5. Stagnant Hypoxia

Another form of hypoxia is *stagnant hypoxia* where there is decreased blood flow, or no wind in the sails – then the blood pressure drops. Stagnant hypoxia comes in two forms: total body, called *shock* and localized, called an *infarction*. If you have a patient in shock you must get him out of shock. You need an ACLS book. (If you don't happen to have one, send for someone who does.) In the book, there is a lovely chapter called *hypotension* with an algorithm that will work you through the problem and get the patient out of shock.

If what you have is a localized infarction, you must re-establish blood flow. You can use balloon angioplasty, clot busters, embolectomy, lasers, diamond tipped roto-rooters, *whatever* – you must get blood flowing again or whatever the artery feeds is going to die. No blood flow, no oxygen delivery, no ATP, no sodium potassium pump, no infrastructure repair, so the cell swells up and becomes dysfunctional. If this goes on long enough, the cell lyses and dies. Enough dead cells, you get a dead patient.

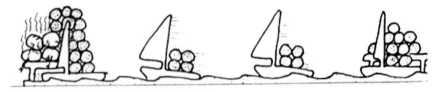

Figure 3-6. Hystotoxic Hypoxia

Our last hypoxia is *hystotoxic hypoxia*. In this form of hypoxia, everything is just fine for delivering the oxygen to the cells, but the cells themselves are dead from cyanide poisoning and can't utilize the oxygen. For example, patients who receive Nipride (nitroprusside) for extended periods of time can die from cyanide poisoning. It turns out that one of the metabolites of Nipride is cyanide. For this reason, we no longer put patients on it for extended periods. We may not always know what we are doing, but we can learn from our mistakes.

Hypoxia is a symptom of a failure to deliver oxygen to the cells where it is used to make ATP. It could be a failure to deliver enough oxygen, a failure of exchange in the lungs, a failure in the transport system, or a failure in the cells' ability to uptake the oxygen. Hypoxia is not a diagnosis; it is a symptom of something else – pneumonia, pulmonary embolus, severe anemia, poor blood flow – something that is compromising the delivery of oxygen into the cells. So, if you have a hypoxic patient, as you are treating the hypoxia you must ask yourself, "Why is this patient hypoxic?" You must find and cure the cause of the hypoxia to make the patient anything more than temporarily better.

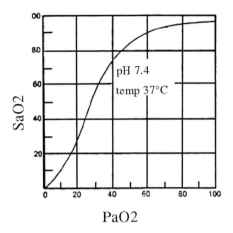

Figure 3-7. Oxy-hemaglobin Disassociation Curve

Have you ever wondered why it is that oxygen clings to hemoglobin in the lungs, but then lets go when the RBC gets out into the tissues? Even if you've never spent a second thinking about it, there are people who have spent their entire careers thinking about it. It has to do with pH. The environment in the lungs is more alkalytic, and oxygen has an affinity for hemaglobin in an alkalytic environment – it grabs right on. Out in the tissues, it is more acidic and the oxygen lets go – it dissociates. All the oxygen-hemoglobin dissociation curve says is that the amount of oxygen available to the patent's tissues depends on the body's pH.

In the good old days, if we were having a code, the first thing we did after we got some lines into the patent was to slam two amps of bicarb into the patent because he had been acidic Every five minutes another amp of bicarb was infused into the patient. We kept working the code, bagging the patient furiously, and got the first blood gas back showing the patient to be alkalytic. We were very pleased with ourselves because the patient wasn't acidic. Well, it turns out that being alkalytic is probably worse than being acidic because less oxygen dissociates from the red blood cell at the tissue level. Your patient needs a normal pH (7.35 to 7.45). So, how much bicarb is given in codes today? Usually, none, though it is a consideration with patients who have a persistent metabolic acidosis that you cannot ventilate into a normal pH. We may not always know what we are doing, but we are capable of learning on a good day.

Assuming 37° C and a normal PaCO2

SaO2	PaO2 @ pH 7.3	PaO2 @ pH 7.4	PaO2 @ pH 7.5
97	101	92	84
96	89	82	74
95	82	76	68
94	76	70	61
93	72	66	60
92	68	62	57
91	64	60	54
90	60	58	51
88	59	54	49
86	56	51	47

Figure 3-8. SaO2 – PaO2 Comparison Chart

The above chart is a comparison between O2 saturation readings and their corresponding arterial blood gas oxygen (PO2) values. There are three PO2s – one with a normal pH, one with an acidic pH, and one with an alkalotic pH. Most of us have an O2 sat of about 97%. If you have a normal pH to go with it, that is a PO2 of 92. A PO2 of 80 to 100 is normal, so 92 is a good number with a lot of wiggle room. If, however, the pH is alkalytic, it is equivalent to a PO2 of 84. If the pH is acidic, it is equivalent to a PO2 of 101.

See how much the pH of the body changes the availability of the body to deliver oxygen to the cells? One would think that making the patient acidic would be a good thing if it increases the dissociation of oxygen at the cellular level. It would if that were all you were concerned with, but remember you must also bind the oxygen to the red blood cell in the first place and that requires an alkalotic environment in the lungs. Your patient needs a normal pH for the system to work correctly. However, in a time of slow blood flow and shock, oxygen is released more quickly from the hemoglobin molecule. Another one of those nice compensatory mechanisms trying to keep you alive.

We frequently begin putting oxygen on patients with an O2 sat of 92. That corresponds to a PO2 of 62 -- if there is a normal pH. It's even worse if there isn't. 80 to 100 is a normal PO2. Why would you let someone get this low before putting oxygen on him? Is there any group of patients for whom this could be a good number? Sure. For elderly people dying of heart and lung disease, this could be the best they have been in six weeks. When you look at numbers, there is no such thing as a right or "normal" number. It always depends on who the patient is. For someone with end-stage lung disease, a sat of 92 could be wonderful.

After a while, we begin to think that normals for whatever kind of patient we take care of the most are normals for everyone. But they aren't. They are only normal for that particular kind of patient.

Some of the most common patients in a hospital today are sick old people dying of heart and lung disease. A few months of taking care of these patients and you begin to think that their normals are normal for the entire patient population. Be careful. Don't extrapolate normals from this group to any other group – they don't fit.

A high school football player was admitted to the hospital with a ruptured appendix. He had peritonitis, so the nurses recognized that atelectasis would be a real problem for this patient. To counter this problem, the nurses got out an incentive spirometer and earnestly went to work on this patient's lungs. He was pulling a liter and a half on the spirometer! The nurses were used to patients pulling 700 cc, 850 cc. They were amazed and gratified at their patient's progress until day three post-op when the morning's chest X-ray showed massive atelectasis! "But why?" they asked. The high school football player should have been pulling two and a half liters! The one and a half liters was a sub-maximal effort for a teenaged athlete, but to the nurses used to sick old people with bad hearts and bad lungs, it looked wonderful. Always consider the patient! Who is this person? What is *his* normal? What are *his* reserves?

Numerous changes happen in your body as you get older. If you are over 30 years old (and if you aren't, this is what you will get on your thirtieth birthday), speed of conduction in the AV node of your heart will start to slow down – so that by the time you are a little old lady or little old man you could possibly have a first degree AV block show up on your EKG and it could possibly be normal for you. Contractility of your heart and oxygen binding capacity will begin to decrease yearly (which is why your exercise capacity has dropped off) so that by the time you are a little old lady or little old man *and are* sedentary you could have a low oxygen saturation and be normal – for you. Being sedentary is a crucial component.

Your body is a communistic enterprise; cells take only what they need to work at an optimum level. When the cells don't take, the body down regulates. Consider these questions: when you go to sleep, does your heartbeat go up or down? What about your blood pressure? Respiratory rate? Oxygen saturation? All go down because the body doesn't need them.

What if you had an 80 year old marathon runner – would you expect to see a low O2 sat? Of course not. If the patient walked the dog for a mile a day or was out puttering in the garden or garage, would you expect to see a low O2 sat? What about the nursing home resident who spends the entire day restlessly wandering the halls trying to figure out how to get out? No. You have to be sedentary to have a low O2 sat (assuming nothing else is causing it).

But who do we see most in our hospitals and care facilities? Little, old, sedentary people in the last years of their lives, dying of heart and lung disease. Their "normals" are not normal for the general population. If I were in your hospital with an O2 sat of 92%, I'd hope that you would please come see why I am not breathing. (I should never have an O2 sat of 92% unless I am in trouble.) Whereas for the little lady with the heart and lung disease, this could be the best she has been in the last week. You have to know who your patient is.

Well, if a 92% O2 sat is so bad, where did the number come from? From the oxygen hemoglobin dissociation curve. See where the top of the curve flattens out at about a 92% (figure 15)? That is the minimum amount of oxygen needed to run the body. But earlier, I said 80 to 100 was a normal PO2 – an 80 PO2 corresponds to a 95% oxygen saturation. Which means that, well, healthy people should never have an oxygen saturation of less than 95%. The oxygen saturation of 92% might be OK in some patients, but consider who you are letting go that low, and remember that every big and little thing in the body requires ATP as an energy source and that it is made of *oxygen* and glucose. An hypoxic patient means a dysfunctional *everything*, including the cardiac action potential.

Patients with respiratory diseases can tolerate lower O2 sats because they are sedentary in their hospital beds. Conversely, if you can't get enough oxygen delivered to a patient's tissues, one thing you can do is to sedate – or to paralyze – the ventilated patient to decrease the cellular demand for oxygen. Movement requires oxygen that could be used for other things.

A 50-year-old man who runs his own business is about to be admitted to the hospital for minor abdominal surgery. On the day of admission, he walks in with an oxygen saturation of 97% – exactly what you would expect from a healthy 50-year-old non-smoker without heart or lung disease. The night of surgery, he requires six liters of oxygen to keep his oxygen saturation up to 92%. The next morning, he's out of bed sitting in a chair and his O2 sat goes back up to 97%. The next night, he lays down and the O2 sat drops back to 92%. The nurses put oxygen on him just as they should. The next morning on rounds, he is sitting up and the O2 saturation returns to 97%. The doctor tells the nurse to stop putting oxygen on the patient at night – a person's oxygen saturation drops at night and besides, the patient looks fine to him.

The next night, the patient lies down and his oxygen saturation again falls to 92%. The nurse does not put oxygen on the patient because of the conversation with the doctor that morning. The patient is also noted to have sleep apnea and had a morphine PCA. Midnight, his saturation is 92%; 0200 it is 92%, 0400 it is

92% and on 7 am rounds, he is found dead with his saturation of 92%. *No one ever asked why* this man's saturation dropped so low whenever he lay down.

Because the patient died unexpectedly, an autopsy was done. This is how we found out exactly what was wrong with him. At the time of his death, his I&O was seven liters up. You might be asking, "Couldn't you see it in his legs or hear it in his lungs?" Someone can put a tremendous amount of fluid into the interstitial spaces around the cells before it ever appears as ankle edema or in the lungs as crackles. In this case, they did hear something: on the last day of this man's life; the staff charted trace ankle edema and distant heart sounds. Remember, this was a big, healthy man. He had a lot of room to put fluid around his cells.

This patient's lungs weighed twice what they should have and he had a new onset pneumonia. There wasn't any exudate in his lungs yet for the staff to hear rattling around, but the alveolar surface was inflamed, so it was more difficult for oxygen to pass through. So, this patient had big, boggy lungs and an inflamed alveolar surface – two factors impeding the passage of oxygen out of the lungs into the circulatory system.

When he was upright, he pooled blood in his extremities. When he lay down, the pooled blood rejoined the circulation, giving him an early cardiogenic pulmonary edema. Add a little sleep apnea and you have a recipe for disaster. Does your hospital have a sleep apnea protocol for patients? If not, they sure need one. Sleep apnea in post-operative patients is a leading cause of death. Treat sleep apnea! And, please don't hesitate to put oxygen on patients if, in your opinion, they need it. The doctor isn't there looking at the patient. You are. Use your best judgment!

Blood Gasses Beyond the Numbers

There are two things of primary importance on a blood gas. There are more things to be seen on the ABG, but we are going to consider the two most important – acid base balance and oxygenation. The acid base balance is the balance between the acid and the base in our bodies. The principal acid is the CO_2 and the main base is our bicarbonate. The balance between the two of them gives the body its pH, which should be 7.35 to 7.45. If the number is larger than 7.4, it is called an alkalosis; if the number is less than 7.35, it is an acidosis.

Next, we look at the PCO_2, the acid load. The value should be 35 to 45. If there is an imbalance in the CO_2, we say there is a respiratory problem. The bicarbonate should be 22 to 26. If there is an imbalance in the bicarbonate, we say the patient has a metabolic problem. Oxygenation is represented by the PO_2, which should be 80 to 100.

This is a good time to talk about oxygenation and O_2 saturation. Oxygen delivery to the cells depends on much more than the saturation of the red blood cells. If you have two red blood cells and both are maximally oxygenated, the O_2 sat will read 100%. It is nice that both are carrying as much oxygen as possible, but it is nowhere near enough to meet the metabolic needs of the body. Delivering oxygen to the body's cells depends on the number of red blood cells, their quality, availability of oxygen, pH of the body, hormones, metabolic conditions and blood flow. Percent of oxygen saturation is just one piece of the puzzle, not the whole picture. Look at your patient – not numbers on a machine!

In the following blood gasses we are going to evaluate numbers, but also
ask ourselves what could be causing this situation and what steps we need to do to rectify it.

pH	7.52
PCO2	35.0
Bicarbonate	28.0
PO2	117

The pH is 7.52, which is greater than 7.45, giving the patient an alkalosis. The CO_2 of 35.0 is the lower end of normal, but the bicarbonate of 28 is high, so our patient has a metabolic problem. It is a metabolic alkalosis, because the pH is greater than 7.45 and the imbalance occurs in the bicarbonate, not the PCO_2.

The patient's PO2 is 117. We would like to know if this patient is on oxygen or not. I have wondered for years how high a person could run their PO2 by hyperventilating on room air. The answer is about 110, although I have heard of a young DKA patient who hyperventilated himself into the 120s on room air with his Kussmal's respirations. There is always someone who can do it better than anyone else.

This patient has a PO2 of 117 – is he on oxygen? Most likely. OK, how much oxygen? You can't make any judgments about his ability to oxygenate himself until you know how much he is on. Maybe he has 2 liters of oxygen going, giving him a PO2 of 117. That is one piece of information. What if he has 100% oxygen going, giving him a PO2 of 117? That is another piece of information.

You can't make any judgments about the patient's ability to oxygenate himself until you know the inspired oxygen (FiO2). How much should a patient's PO2 change when the FiO2 is changed? The PO2 should be about 3-4 times what the FiO2 is. For example, if you put a patient on 100% oxygen, you should see a PO2 of be between 300 and 400. If you don't, you have an hypoxic patient, because he is not oxygenating as well as expected. This is a way of seeing hypoxia early in the acute lung injury patient before he becomes an acute respiratory distress patient.

"*But,*" you say, "*a PO2 of 80 to 100 is normal and 117 is above normal. How can the patient be hypoxic?*" It is a matter of what you have versus what is expected. The ration of FiO2 to PO2 is off; something is happening. This is another early sign of impending doom. Patients shouldn't need oxygen to have normal oxygenation. "*It's only 2 liters,*" you say. But it shouldn't be anything. Our lungs have tremendous reserve capability. If you need any oxygen at all to have a "normal" PO2, you have a problem.

Let's look at the concept of *Normal Values*. Normal for whom? People doing what? Normal for well, healthy individuals breathing room air with a normal respiratory rate under normal conditions – such as someone who's sitting in front of a TV set. These are not the same normals experienced by a person who is having an MI, in septic shock, or has some other acute life-threatening event. "Normal" applies to people *without* multiple problems.

As we work the rest of the ABGs, we will begin to question the viability of normal. Remember, *everything always* depends.

pH	7.18
PCO2	56.0
Bicarbonate	22.0
PO2	41.0

In this gas, we have a pH of 7.18 which is low, a PCO2 of 56 which is high, and a bicarbonate that is the bottom end of normal. An acidic pH and an abnormal PCO2 give us a respiratory acidosis. One of the things you can tell from a blood gas is how long the event has been going on. You cannot walk around with an abnormal pH. This pH is out of sync because of the large acid (CO2) load. To compensate for this, the body will retain a lot of the base bicarbonate and swing the pH back to normal. The body retains the bicarbonate in the kidneys, which can take days. Looking at this ABG, is this an acute or chronic situation? Has the body had days to retain bicarbonate, compensate for the huge acid load and return the pH to normal? No, so this is an acute respiratory acidosis and *not* something that has been going on for days.

The PO2 is 41. What is this patient not doing? He's not breathing, and I sincerely hope you noticed it before the gas came back! You have a patient who is acutely not breathing and he needs your help. Some stimulation, a few drugs, an ET tube – *something*, or he is going to be dead.

Speaking of dead, how do you get that way? From a lethal dysrhythmia. What caused this patient's lethal dysrhythmia? Both the pH and hypoxia. He has two of the four things that can make you dead – pH, electrolytes, glucose and oxygen. This patient is screaming towards a lethal dysrhythmia just as fast as he can by two separate pathways and if you don't oxygenate and perfuse at the same time to keep his pH normal, his electrolytes balanced, and O2 and glucose inside the cell being used to make ATP, he will be successful.

pH	7.37
PCO2	55.0
Bicarbonate	31.0
PO2	65

In this gas we have a normal pH, a high PCO2, and high bicarbonate. This is a respiratory acidosis as seen by the high CO2, but the pH is normal because this patient has had days to retain bicarbonate in his kidneys and swing his pH back to normal. This is, therefore, a patient who is used to having his PCO2 high – a CO2 retaining COPDer. He retains bicarbonate and swings his pH back to normal, because you must have a normal pH for the cells to function properly, and life is about appropriately functioning cells.

This patient is a CO2 retaining COPDer. We need to differentiate the Retainer from the average COPDer. In the great category of COPD, there is a small subcategory called retainers. They are few in number when compared to the whole because CO2 exchanges across the membrane in the lungs 20 times faster than oxygen does. By the time someone is retaining CO2, they have destroyed so much of their lung tissue that they will, 1) never have a normal PO2, and 2) not live very long. They do, however, flood into our hospitals the last few years of their lives, making it seem that all COPDers are also retainers. Not true, it can just seem so by looking at our patient populations.

In this ABG, the patient has a PO2 of 65. A PO2 of 80 – 100 is normal. Shall we turn up the FiO2? Is our patient a CO2 retaining COPDer? Yes, you can see it with the high CO2 and the normal pH. This means the condition had been present for the days required to retain bicarb in the kidneys and swing the pH back to normal.

What causes a CO2 retaining COPDers only drive to breathe? We have always taught you the hypoxic drive theory stating that you and I have two drives to breathe. One, if our PCO2 goes up we breathe faster and two, if our PO2 goes down we breathe faster. If you have a chronically high PCO2, you blunt the CO2 receptors and they don't respond anymore. Now your only drive to breathe is hypoxia. The hypoxic drive theory is currently under debate, but what happens to the patient if he gets too much oxygen is not under debate. He lays down, goes to sleep, and never wakes up again. The mechanism of the dysfunction is under debate. Is it because the oxygen suppressed the drive to breathe, or is it because giving the patient oxygen changed blood flow patterns through the lungs, then he picked up CO_2 that was already present and moved it into the circulatory system? You ask if it makes a difference. Yes, it does.

If a patient is hypoxic, absolutely nothing requiring ATP to function is working right. This includes the action potential. People who live with chronic hypoxia are similar to people with chronic severe pain in the sense that one more little pinprick will send them right over the edge. The chronically hypoxic patient has learned to live with a certain level of hypoxia; you take away just a little bit of oxygen in his body and he panics. When he panics, the heart rate and blood pressure goes up, the workload of the heart increases, there isn't enough oxygen to make ATP and repolarize the action potential and there goes the lethal dysrythmia.

You do not want these people to panic, but we don't want to give them too much oxygen, either, as the hypoxic drive theory has not been disproven; it's just under debate. This means that you need to make sure your retainer stays hypoxic. The question is, how hypoxic do they need to be? You don't want your patient to be any more hypoxic than he absolutely has to be, because ATP runs everything in the body and ATP requires oxygen. Nothing is functioning properly in the body of a hypoxic patient.

The mistake we make with the ABGs for a CO_2 retainer is that we look at the PO2 of 65 and say, "Oh, he's a retainer. He needs to be hypoxic so leave him alone." Always take the ABG results to the bedside and see how the patient is doing with those numbers. If he is playing cards with his wife, is this a good number for him? If he is confused, weak, and hostile is this a good PO2 for him? It always depends on how the patient is doing with the numbers that determines if that number is good for him. Maybe he wants his PO2 a little closer to 70 or 75 – never normal – but maybe he could use half, one, or maybe 2 liters FiO2 for optimal functioning.

Make no decisions from a piece of paper; always go see how the patient is doing with these numbers.

Don't make these patients struggle to breathe any more than they absolutely have to. The amount of stress and exercise that can be endured is directly related to the amount of oxygen available to make ATP. Remember, the brain uses ATP to fire neurons. Look for changes in mentation, cognitive ability and irritability when determining where to set the flow meter.

pH	7.53
PCO2	26.0
Bicarbonate	22.0
PO2	162

This gas shows a patient with a high pH, a low PCO2 and normal bicarbonate. This represents a respiratory alkalosis because the PCO2 is low and therefore responsible for the high pH. People with respiratory alkalosis are most frequently doing what? Hyperventilating. The most common cause of hyperventilating is not anxiety, nor is it pain – it is hypoxia. Hypoxia will make a patient very anxious, especially if the people around them are saying stupid things like "*Lay down! Slow your breathing down!*" At this point, patients know these people don't have a clue what is wrong with them and they aren't paying attention.

What gender of patient is most likely to get an anxiety attack diagnosis? Women. By far, women are more likely to be given an anxiety attack diagnosis. If you take nothing else away from this whole book, the most important piece of knowledge I want you to remember is that the number one cause of hyperventilation is hypoxia. Make sure the patient isn't hypoxic first before giving her a psychological diagnosis.

This patient has a PO2 of 162. Is hypoxia the cause of his hyperventilation? No, he is not hypoxic, so that cannot be a cause of this patient's hyperventilation.

You may also see values like this with an acute cardiac event. You have a patient whose heart isn't pumping as well as it should and therefore isn't delivering oxygen to the tissues in adequate amounts. The tissues become hypoxic and send a chemical message to the pneumotaxic center in the brain requesting the person to breathe faster. Because the lungs are normal, the increase in respiration causes the patient to blow off CO_2 with the resultant respiratory alkalosis.

Our patient has a PO_2 of 162. Our normal PO_2 is 80 – 100. Should we turn the FiO_2 down? Make no judgments about what to do with a gas until you know the circumstances. Is this patient in the midst of a cardiac event? If he is, are you going to turn his oxygen down? Of course not; you would likely precipitate his lethal dysrhythmia and death. Circumstances are crucial in the decision-making process. Remember, normals are normal for well, healthy people under normal circumstances , not for people in the throes of a cardiac crisis. You give the patient all the oxygen he needs to help him through the event, *then* you turn the oxygen down.

This patient has a PO_2 of 162. Can you hyperventilate yourself to a PO_2 of 162? No. Someone has put oxygen on this patient. Let's say that someone was you and let's say he is having an MI. Why do you put oxygen on someone having an MI? So they will have good tissue perfusion and won't go anaerobic and start cranking out lactic acid? Sure, you bet. But what has to happen first? A heartbeat. And what causes the heart to contract? The action potential – the electrical request for squeeze. The first thing that has to happen is the repolarization of the last action potential to get ready for the next heartbeat to come down -- that will require oxygen to make ATP.

The reason you put oxygen on a patient having an MI (or any other emergency for that matter) is to help them repolarize their action potential. Sometimes people say, "Why did you put oxygen on him?" To which you reply, "To make sure he repolarized his action potential!" It usually shuts them right up. Remember, you don't have to be smart, you just need to understand a few concepts; people will think you are smart, and that is all that counts.

Ph	7.10
PCO2	35.0
Bicarbonate	11.0
PO2	338

The acidic pH in this gas is being caused by a very low bicarbonate level and is therefore called a metabolic acidosis. Is it acute or chronic? If the pH is still out of whack, then it is acute. Things that can cause a metabolic acidosis include diabetic keto acidosis and ion gap acidosis form an electrolyte imbalance. But by far the largest number of metabolic acidosis cases are caused by lactic acidosis: because of a failure to oxygenate, a failure to perfuse, or a failure to oxygenate and perfuse at the same time.

Our patient has a PO2 of 338. Can we all agree to turn his FiO2 down? Is he well and healthy, or is he in crisis? We know he is in crisis from looking at the pH. The most likely thing to have caused the pH to be so low is a lactic acidosis from a failure to oxygenate, a failure to perfuse, or a failure to oxygenate and perfuse. We see his oxygenation is good with a PO2 of 338. How much oxygen is being inspired on this patient? This one you can tell – 100% oxygen because the PO2 is more than three times the FiO2. Since there is nothing wrong with this patient's lungs, let's put our money on failure to perfuse due to shock for some reason. If this patient has a low blood pressure, are you going to turn his FiO2 down? Of course not; you would precipitate his lethal dysrhythmia secondary to poor perfusion into the myocardium, and a failure to repolarize his action potential. Always ask yourself what the circumstances are surrounding the values. People in shock are not well and healthy – normals don't apply. In this case, we are going to make this patient better, get him out of crisis, stabilize him, and *then* turn his oxygen down.

pH	7.46
PCO2	32.0
Bicarbonate	22.0
PO2	69.0

A young student nurse (this is relevant because student nurses are well known for developing every disease they read about in their textbooks) went into the ER complaining of shortness of breath, chest discomfort, and sudden anxiety while studying for the next day's test The ER shot a chest X-ray and didn't see anything abnormal; drew a blood gas which showed classic hyperventilation with a low CO2, but you could look at her and tell she was hyperventilating. So, they gave her the diagnosis of anxiety attack secondary to tomorrow's big test and sent her back to the dorm.

The student felt something was really wrong inside, so she called her mother seeking advice. The mother called the family physician who instructed the mother to tell the daughter to go back to the ER immediately and tell the physician that her family has a hyper coagulable syndrome, causing them to make clots at the drop of a hat. Upon further workup, it was found that this young woman had thrown a pulmonary embolus so huge it occluded one entire lung. Because she was so young and so healthy she was able to hyperventilate herself into an almost normal gas in the face of a catastrophic event.

If this young woman had never received any care for her PE, what probably would have happened to her? Died? Not necessarily. You and I throw PEs all the time. We have 80,000 miles of blood vessels in our bodies. We make clots in them all the time. They break off and travel to the lungs where they get stuck in the pulmonary vasculature. Size matters. The body comes along with its own anti-thrombin III, and opens the vessel back up. If you put a patient with PEs – lets say on heparin – does the heparin get rid of the PE? No. Then what is it there for? To keep the clot you have from getting any bigger (to occlude the lumen they are in) and keep the patient from making new ones. So what gets rid of the PE? The patient's own anti-thrombin III.

Considering how young and healthy this woman was, she might have been able to dissolve her PE in time. But when she threw her next PE, then went back into the ER, she had a diagnosis of "anxiety attack" on her ER record. Do you even think they would have shot a chest X-ray? Speaking of which, can you see a PE on a chest X-ray? No, you can't. You can get some hints it might be there, but the younger and healthier the patient is, the less likely those hints are to be there.

So, the number one cause of hyperventilation is what? Hypoxia. This student nurse survived her PE, bit I was told of another student nurse who went into the ED with PEs and was told she was having an anxiety attack. She died from her PEs.

In the above gas, the pH is slightly alkalotic, but barely so. However, you can't be a little alkalotic any more than you can be a little pregnant. You either are or you aren't. 7.45 is normal; 7.46 is alkalytic. We can see that the cause for the pH is the low PCO_2 resulting in a rather mild respiratory alkalosis. The patient is breathing rapidly enough to blow off CO_2. What is the most common cause of hyperventilation? Hypoxia. Is this patient hypoxic? The PO_2 is 69. Earlier, on a previous gas I stated that the PO_2 of 65 might be a good number for that patient. Is there any way that this PO_2 of 69 is OK for this patient? No. How can you tell? Because it is an acute situation. The bicarbonate is normal, the pH is abnormal, and there hasn't been time for compensation. This is a patient with an acute hypoxic event. But the gas is rather unremarkable, isn't it? No, not at all. This gas screams acute hypoxic event in a person with good compensatory mechanisms.

The younger and healthier you are the more likely you are to be able to hyperventilate yourself into a fairly normal gas. The older and sicker you are, the quicker you crash. Remember, the number one cause of hyperventilation is hypoxia and that hypoxia makes you very anxious. You shouldn't have to hyperventilate to give yourself a "normal" PO_2.

pH	7.06
PCO_2	40.3
Bicarbonate	1.4
PO_2	86.0

This patient has a very acidic pH caused by the very low

bicarbonate. It has happened quickly and his PCO2 isn't able to respond and bring the pH back to normal. We have an acute metabolic acidosis. The PO2 is 86; 80 to 100 is normal. Do you want to change the FiO2? Turn it up, maybe? Is this patient in crisis? Yes. How do you know? Look at the pH. This patient is getting ready to have his lethal dysrhythmia caused by the severe acidosis. Abnormal pH is one of the four things that can lead to a lethal dysrhythmia and this is a very abnormal pH. What is the most common cause of a metabolic acidosis? Lactic acidosis caused by a failure to oxygenate, a failure to perfuse, or a failure to oxygenate and perfuse at the same time.

Is this patient a failure to oxygenate? He has a PO2 of 86. Isn't that normal? It depends on how much oxygen is being inspired. If this patient is on 100% oxygen with a PO2 of 86, he is a flat-out failure to oxygenate. His PO2 should be greater than 300. The most likely thing to have caused this patient to be so incredibly acidic is shock. If you have a patient in shock and you don't have them on 100% oxygen, I hope your malpractice insurance is all paid up because that is a huge mistake.

Does this gas belong to a well, healthy individual? Do normals apply in this acute crisis? The most likely thing causing this acidosis is a low blood pressure. If this patient is in shock, do you want him to be left with a normal PO2? No. You want to shove the FiO2 just as high as you can get it, make the patient all better, then turn the oxygen down after you have corrected the problem and stabilized the patient. Having to run a code will totally ruin your day.

pH	7.35
PCO2	60.0
Bicarbonate	34.0
PO2	101.0

In this gas, two abnormals make a normal. There is a high PCO2 representing a large acid load and a high bicarbonate representing a large base load. The two of them compensate for each other and result in a normal pH. This is another gas belonging to a CO2 retaining COPDer. The PCO2 is high at 60 and the chronic component is seen in the time required for the kidney to retain bicarbonate and swing the pH back to normal. This patient is used to having his CO2 up and has nicely balanced himself.

Which came first, the high CO2 or the high bicarb? You can tell because the body never overcompensates. When it gets the pH into the normal range it stops compensating, so whichever the pH is closest to (acidotic or alkalotic) points to the original problem. This pH is closest to an acidic condition; therefore, the CO2 acid load was the original problem. What if the pH had been 7.44; where would the problem have started? Right, the base, the bicarbonate.

This patient has a PO2 of 101. Normal is 80 to 100. Do you want to change his rate of inspired oxygen? Does it depend on how he is doing with these numbers? He's doing great. He's watching Millionaire Survivor Apprentice Bachelorette on TV and he is laughing and having a good time. Do you want to turn his oxygen down? Yes, absolutely.

Is this patient a CO2 retaining COPDer? Absolutely. That means that his only drive to breathe might be hypoxia, and he is not hypoxic with a PO2 of 101.

I said he was doing fine, and he is right now, but CO2 narcosis usually takes hours. Hypoxia kills in seconds to minutes. Some retainers will crash and burn quickly, but most spend hours going into CO2 narcosis.

A CO2 retaining COPDer in the last year of her life came into the hospital to be intubated, cleaned out, and set right about once a month. On this particular day, she called 911, but when the paramedics got there, they didn't need to intubate her. She was in crisis, so they gave her 100% oxygen, which was exactly the right thing to do. They transported her to the ER, where she got further treatment but did not need intubation. The 100% oxygen was still flowing.

The ER decided after treatment that not only did they to need to intubate her, she did not require the ICU either, so they called for a room on the floor. The high flow oxygen was still going. Hours later, she arrived on the floor with her high flow oxygen still going. She was admitted, the nurse brought her lunch, she ate, turned over, and went to sleep. She awakened several hours later in the ICU on a ventilator with a PCO2 of 120. You cannot leave the high flow oxygen on.

How Much Oxygen Should You Give a CO2 Retaining COPDer in Crisis?

In the good old days after we had just learned that there was such a thing as a CO2 retaining COPDer, we were taught that if you gave them too much oxygen they lay down, went to sleep, and didn't wake up again. This was an adverse outcome. The word went out that all COPDers could have 2 liters of oxygen and *no more than 2* liters FiO2, no matter what was going on. The educational campaign was massive and complete. Everyone heard that COPDers were to be limited to 2 liters of oxygen – no more – and we all complied.

Then someone came along and did a study, and found that if you limit these patients to 2 liters of oxygen at the time of the exacerbation of their COPD, they died in large numbers from lethal dysrythmias because they could not repolarize their action potentials. So then the word went out that COPDers could have all the oxygen they needed when they were in crisis. Unfortunately, the group that put out the 2 liter rule had a much better educational campaign than the group trying to take it back. What we are left with is a great deal of confusion in some circles about how much oxygen you should give a CO2 retaining COPDer – particularly among older nurses who were around for the indoctrination. Since we train the new nurses, we have managed to confuse everyone about how much oxygen to give a CO2 retaining COPDer *in crisis*.

Remember that the only patients who have trouble with oxygen are CO2 retaining COPDers. The average COPDer has no trouble with oxygen. Remember also, that we are talking about the short run – the patient in crisis. On top of his COPD, this patient also has fluid overload, pneumonia, an asthma attack or something else that is exacerbating his lung disease. His life is in danger. What is he going to die from? A lethal dysrhythmia caused by an abnormal pH, an imbalance in his electrolytes, or not having oxygen and glucose in the cells being used to make ATP.

Let's look at how much oxygen we are saying today you should give a CO_2 retaining COPDer in crisis – and only if they are in crisis. We have a patient who is a genuine CO_2 retaining COPDer. On a good day, he has a PO2 of 75. It will never be normal because he is a retainer and his disease has destroyed a great deal of his lung tissue. He has had an exacerbation of his COPD and his PO2 drops to 60. Does he have a drive to breathe? Is he hypoxic? You bet. He is severely hypoxic. Since you understand about ATP formation and the action potential, you give him 100% oxygen because you don't want him to die from a lethal dysrhythmia, and he thanks you. He's not ready to go just yet.

We keep working on him and the next gas comes back with a PO2 of 65. Does he have a drive to breathe? Is he hypoxic? Yes, he is. We keep working and the next gas has a PO2 of 68. Does he have a drive to breathe? Sure, he's still hypoxic for him. Next gas the PO2 is 72. Does he have a drive to breathe? Yes. On the next gas, the PO2 is 76. Does he have a drive to breathe? No, he has exceeded his normal PO2 of 75. Actually, you needed to start paying attention to him when the PO2 was 72. But from the 60 all the way to 72, the patient needed 100% oxygen to keep from dying from a lethal dysrhythmia. From 72 to 75, it depends on what he is normally on. If he is normally on 2 liters, he gets 4 liters, if he normally is on room air he gets 2 liters and when he hits his normal PO2, it is whatever he normally is on ... whether that be room air, half a liter, 2 liters, whatever. But, if you limit him to 2 liters of oxygen at the time of the exacerbation of his COPD when he is so horribly hypoxic, he is likely to not survive the event.

When you observe the behavior of patients, you can get some clues as to the status of their oxygenation. People who are hypoxic are confused, restless, agitated, and combative. Please – never sedate anyone for being confused, restless, agitated or combative until you can prove that this particular episode of confused, restless, agitated and combative behavior is not being driven by hypoxia. Don't forget to document it.

Let's say you have two patients. One is a raving lunatic, the other a sweet little old lady who sundowns at 7 pm every night. It is now 7:15 pm and both of these patient s are confused, restless, agitated, and combative. Could they have just thrown a pulmonary embolus, developed pneumonia, be having an MI? Absolutely. So always make sure the patient's behavior isn't being driven by hypoxia before you sedate them. Sedating hypoxic patients,can kill them.

If confused, restless, agitated, combative is the sign of hypoxia, what is the sign of CO2 narcosis (high CO2)? The opposite; a somnolent patient, the patient you cannot get to wake up, which is a 180° difference from the restless hypoxic patient. Surely, now that you know this, you will not have any trouble trying to determine the difference between the hypoxic and somnolent patient's oxygen needs. Unfortunately, it isn't always that easy. Patients haven't always read this book and sometimes they don't know how to act when they present themselves to you. You look at the patient and say, "I don't know. He's not clearly this and he's not clearly that. What do I do?" You put *oxygen* on the patient for three very good reasons. 1) CO2 narcosis *usually* takes hours; hypoxia kills in seconds to minutes, 2) it is harder to run a hypoxic code than it is to deal with a somnolent patient, and 3) you may not get your patient back from the hypoxic code, but you can always take the oxygen off. Putting oxygen on the patient buys you time – time for the team to show up; time for the blood gas to come back; time for someone who knows this patient to show up.

So, what liter flow should we start with? Two liters? What did I say about the 2 liter rule? We have a patient in trouble, not sitting and watching TV. Start with 4-5 liters FiO2. If there is any trouble in the blood pressure, go immediately to 100% oxygen. We must repolarize the action potential. "On a CO2 retaining COPDer," you ask? Yes! They have action potentials, too.

Let's say we have the genuine article, a CO2 retaining COPDer having an MI. You put 5 liters of oxygen on him because I told you to. He then extends the MI and you are now having trouble with his blood pressure. You shove him up to 100% oxygen because I told you to, and his CO2 shoots up and you have to intubate and ventilate him. Have you done a bad thing by giving him all that oxygen? No. He is alive to be intubated. What if you had limited him to 2 liters FiO2 at the time he extended his MI. What would've happened had you not done this? He'd have likely been dead from a lethal dysrythmia. You must repolarize the action potential. While you're doing this, please try to wash the 2 liter rule out of your brain. (Even if you didn't say it, I know you were probably thinking it.)

Key Components to Chapter 3

1. Normal ABG numbers imply a well, healthy individual, breathing room air, with a normal respiratory rate.
2. You have to know what a normal number is for this patient.
3. 92% sat is NOT the bottom end of normal. 95% sat is. Know the patient.
4. Women are most often given the diagnosis of "anxiety attack" and turned away from the health care system.
5. The number one cause of hyperventilation is hypoxia.
6. Hypoxia will make you very anxious from the sympathetic stimulation it causes.
7. The most common cause of a metabolic acidosis is lactic acidosis

Chapter 4
The Cardiac Cycle

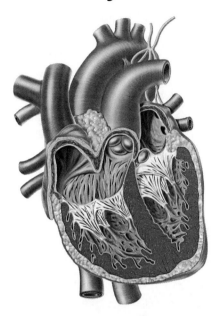

Figure 4-1. Anatomy of the Human Heart

When the heart squeezes, it uses ATP as an energy source – of which there is a finite, not infinite amount. So, when the heart squeezes, you want the blood to go out in the direction that you want it to, not back in the direction that it came from. That is wasted energy. To direct the blood flow in the direction that you want it to go, the heart is equipped with a series of valves. The mitral and tricuspid valves are just tissue paper thin leaflets with little structure. The leaflets are attached via chordae tendineae (like parachute harnesses) to a structure called a papillary muscle that rises up out of the floor of the myocardium. When the heart contracts, the blood is sent backward with the same force it is pushed out the way you want it to go, but the papillary muscle also contracts and pulls the valve leaflets down nice and tight. That is what ensures the blood is forced out the right way.

These papillary muscles are made of cells with sodium – potassium – ATP pumps that need to be run, infrastructure that needs to be repaired, and internal operations that need to be performed. The requirements for all of these functions are brought into the papillary muscle cells by the perfusion into the myocardium. If you have an area of the heart that is ischemic, it will not squeeze as well as the rest of the heart. If that ischemia includes a papillary muscle, it will not pull down as tightly as the other papillary muscles. What would that sound like in your stethoscope? A murmur.

A new onset murmur should be considered a medical emergency until proven otherwise. If a papillary muscle is ischemic, it becomes dysfunctional, doesn't pull tight enough, and results in a murmur. If the ischemia goes on long enough or is severe enough, the patient can rupture that papillary muscle. Now you have a valve leaflet blowing in the breeze. This occurs most often to the mitral valve on the left side of the heart where the pressures are higher. When this happens, only half the blood goes out the aorta when the heart contracts. (There goes half your cardiac output.) The other half goes directly back into the patient's lungs giving him an acute, four-plus pulmonary edema. This is a catastrophe your patient probably will not survive. New onset heart murmurs also occur in patients tearing their aorta down into their aortic valve or trying to eat a hole through the septum of their heart. These are all medical emergencies.

Time is of the essence. Once the papillary muscle is ruptured or the aorta or septum have deteriorated, the horse is out of the barn. The problem needs to be detected before the rupture or tear. You hear the problem coming with a new onset murmur. If you put your stethoscope on a patient's chest and you hear a murmur that no one ever heard before, get other people in the room to listen. If you are the only nurse around, this is an excellent time to call your Rapid Response Team.

This patient needs help. Whether the open heart surgery is one floor up, 30 miles down the road in an ambulance, or over the hills in a helicopter, it takes time. Time to clean a room, or prime the pump, or get the team in from home, it takes time. You can buy your patient that time by having an index of suspicion. If you hear something new in that patient's chest, get other people in the room to listen. If it is a new onset heart murmur you may have just saved this patient's life.

Cardiac patients are the kind of patients most likely to rupture a papillary muscle, particularly those having inferior events. But did you know that as many as 30 - 50% of the people having MIs never give us a symptom that we recognize as an MI? This is called *silent* ischemia. It is so prevalent that there is even a *Journal of Silent Ischemia*. This is the person who goes in for his yearly physical, and after the EKG, the doctor asks him when he had his MI. The patient doesn't remember a MI, but he did have a bad case of the flu last June. That was the MI. So, the patient admitted with pneumonia or a small bowel obstruction can also have an undetected MI and papillary muscle rupture by tearing his aorta or destroying the septum of his heart. If you do indeed have a new onset murmur, you need a doctor right now.

If you hear a new onset murmur, get other people involved. Do *not* assume you have made a mistake because no one else had heard it before.

Systole and Diastole

Diastole

During diastole there are three crucial things happening in the heart. The first is the filling of the ventricles. Next is the repolarization of the action potential. If you depolarized, when will you repolarize? Diastole. And, when does the heart muscle itself get its blood supply? When it is squeezing or when it is relaxed? When it is relaxed. The three things that happen during diastole are filling, repolarization, and coronary perfusion.

These three things take time. The problem with tachy dysrythmias is that they take away your time component. There isn't time to properly fill the heart and stroke volume and, thereby cardiac output, drops off. Repolarization can be negatively affected, leading to dysrhythmias, of which some can be fatal. The myocardium itself is poorly perfused and the patient develops deficiencies in myocardial contractility, also known by the medical term "crappy squeeze."

If the patient has poor perfusion into their myocardium, and if that perfusion occurs during diastole, the longer the diastole, the more time there is to get blood into the myocardium. This is why you see doctors slow their patient's heart rates down so much. Part is to decrease the workload of the heart; part is to increase the diastolic filling time.

Have you ever wondered how it is that the blood is pumped from the left heart and manages to make it over to the right heart? "Well," you say, "You shove it from the left heart with a high pressure and it ends up in the right heart with a low pressure." Yes, but no. You do indeed shove it from the left with a high pressure, but you shove it out into the aorta which is a large diameter vessel. As the blood goes down the circulatory tree the vessels get smaller, smaller, and smaller until the capillaries are one-cell thick. Then, the vessels get bigger, bigger, and bigger on the venous side and dump the blood into the right heart. You can't push through something like that. You need a different system of pressures.

If you have an intact column of fluid that meets itself at its ends forming a circle, which is what our cardiovascular system is, it isn't so much that you shove with the high pressure generated in the left heart as you literally suck with the low pressure in the right heart. Maintaining the low pressures in the right heart is crucial to getting the blood to come up and around the cardiovascular circuit. The heart sits in the chest, which is a low pressure system, and when we take in a breath we drop the pressures in the chest and augment blood flow back into the right heart. If anything were to increase the pressures in the chest, it can keep the blood from returning to the heart – things like sucking chest wounds, a tension pneumothorax, PEEP on a ventilator, or pulmonary hypertension. These things raise the pressure in the chest and can overcome the ability of the blood to return to the right heart.

Consider a patient out riding his motorcycle on a beautiful spring day. He gets involved in an accident and is now flying through the air at 30 miles per hour when he sees a stop sign approaching and decides to reach out and grab it. Bad idea. He is now lying on the ground and his blood supply is lying on the ground next to him. He does not have an intact column of fluid. In order to save his life, you must plug the hole, fill him back up, and give him an intact column of fluid.

The next thing our motorcyclist has to have is a distensible heart. When you pour blood into the heart, it has to get bigger. If it doesn't, we have a serious problem, because you cannot get out of the left heart any more than you were able to get into the right heart. Things that would keep you heart from distending are conditions like restrictive cardiomyopathy, restrictive pericarditis, or pressures in the wrong place, as in cardiac tamponade.

An example of restrictive cardiomyopathy is amyloidosis. Once I had a patient whose chest X-ray looked like he had gravel all around his heart. He had a chronic pericardial inflammation into which he put calcium. Calcium does not distend, so he had a restrictive pericarditis.

In cardiac tamponade, there is so much fluid in the pericardial sac surrounding the heart that it pushes up on the walls of the ventricles and they can't distend. It is a matter of pressures in the right places. Sometimes there is nothing wrong with the heart itself for the patient with tamponade; you put a needle into the pericardial sac, withdraw the fluid and the heart works just fine. It is a matter of pressures in the right places.

If you have an intact column of fluid, a distensible heart, and pressures in the right place, you get the first part of diastole: passive filling. The second part of diastole is an active filling. The atria are going to contract, and when they do, they are capable of shoving as much as 30-40% more volume down into the ventricle. This is called the atrial kick. This reserve is part of the sympathetic response – fight or flight. As you are sitting quietly, your atrial kick is giving you little of your total cardiac output – 10-15% – because you don't need it. But, if you should have to jump up and run, it can give you as much as 40% more cardiac output.

What a tremendous reserve. It has been said that a patient in the unit, post-op, septic, on a ventilator requires the same amount of energy as a person continually running four minute miles. If you were running four minute miles, would you want your atrial kick? Of course you would. Dysrhythmias that can take away the p wave that signifies atrial contraction include atrial fibrillation, atrial flutter, junctional, ventricular, and some of the blocks. Any time you don't have one "p" in front of every QRS you have lost the atrial kick and potentially 40% of the total cardiac output.

We spend a lot of time trying to put people back into sinus rhythm these days. In the good old days, if someone went into atrial fibrillation, we didn't spend a lot of time trying to get him out of it. We gave him some digitalis and hoped his atrial fibrillation would get better. Today, we spend a great deal of time and effort trying to get people out of atrial fibrillation. We will shock you, drug you, ablate you – we want you out of atrial fibrillation so you can resume your full cardiac output.

Systole

We've had passive filling and gotten our atrial kick. It is now time for systole. I had a student say to me one time, "*Can you die with a pacemaker in?*" Of course you can. At this point, I realized that I had told the students all about ATP, those four conditions, and the action potential, but what I had forgotten to tell them was that if the four conditions of normal pH, balanced electrolytes, oxygen and glucose inside the cell being used to make ATP are not met in the individual myocardial cell, it will not respond to the electrical request for squeeze. The good stuff comes to the myocardial cells because of coronary circulation. It brings the good stuff in and takes the bad stuff away. If you want good, brisk systole, you must have good, brisk coronary circulation. This is why we spend so much time revascularizing our patients' hearts.

Systole and diastole cycle over 100,000 times a day and it is a miracle it works once.

Cardiac output = heart rate X stroke volume

74

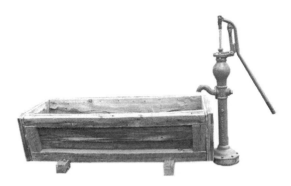

Figure 4-2. Trigger, Trough and Pump

Let's say you and your horse Trigger live in the flat, barren, hot prairie. Trigger has osmoreceptors and an active thirst mechanism; he will need drinks of water just like you do. To supply the water you have a horse trough which you fill with an old fashioned hand-crank pump. These pumps differ from faucets. When you turn a faucet on, the water runs until you turn the faucet off, but with this hand pump, the water only comes out when you push down on the handle. Every time you stroke down on the handle, a certain volume of water comes out, and nothing happens until you push down again. We will call the volume that comes out the *stroke volume* and how fast you push the rate.

Everything is just fine for you and Trigger, until one day you notice that when you push down on the handle, less volume comes out. Trigger considers this to be your personal problem – he wants his horse trough full. How can you keep the trough full if less comes out each time you push down on the handle? That's right; push faster to get the same total volume out.

To detect the source of the problem, you get out your fiber optic scope and snake it down into the well and see that the aquifer is running dry. This requires moving on to Plan B. Plan B is to drill yourself another well directly into your neighbor's aquifer which is brimming over with water. She hates you and is pretty sure this is exactly what you have done. Now, every time you push down on the handle, water gushes out all over the place. If she can see this water everywhere, she will know that you are into her aquifer. How can you keep the horse trough full, but not over flowing? Yes, turn the rate down. Other students have said to get another horse, or a bigger horse trough, or give Lasix to Trigger and he will deposit the water all over the ranch. Those last possibilities represent critical thinking (CT). CT is about possibilities.

Cardiac output equals heart rate times stroke volume, and if anything affects stroke volume, you see a compensatory rise or fall in the heart rate. Stroke volume isn't the only thing affecting heart rate. So do each of the following:

- hypoxia
- sympathetic stimulation (pain, fear, anxiety)
- fever (10 bpm for every degree F of temp above normal),
- drugs
- exercise, and
- metabolic events (myxedema coma, thyroid storm, response to injury, etc.)

You have a post-op patient with a heart rate of 110. Is this a good heart rate on a post-op patient? Maybe is the correct answer. It depends on the company the heart rate keeps. Maybe the patient came out of surgery with a heart rate of 80. That afternoon it went to 90 and that night it was 100, and now this morning it is 110 bpm. Is something going on? What? You don't know, but you do know that heart rate starting to climb represents the body's compensation for hypoxia, fever, sympathetic stimulation, exercise, drugs, and metabolic events.

When we were in school, they taught us the signs of illness, but before the body becomes ill, it tries to compensate. If you can see the signs of compensation, you have an advanced warning that your patient is in trouble. There are three signs of the body is trying to compensate. They are: heart rate starting to climb, respiratory rate starting to climb, and urine output less than it had been before. We will look at the respiratory rate and urine output later, but let's consider heart rate right now. Remember, that it is when compensation fails that we get the signs of illness. Sometimes, devastating events occur to a patient, and later you wonder if you could have been able to see it coming before it overwhelmed you and the patient. Someone did a study on this topic. When patients crash and burn, how long before the crash were the signs there, able to be seen if you only knew what you supposed to be looking for? Eight hours prior to the crash, the signs are there if you know what you are looking for – what you are looking for are signs of compensation in the body. Signs the body is trying to make things better.

So, you *can* see it coming. You see it coming in our post-op patient with a heart rate of 110 by noticing that his heart rate is starting to rise. By the time the heart rate reaches 150, Helen Keller could probably see a problem, but you want to catch it early. And the only way to do so is to look at trends. Without looking at trends, there is no way you will know if the heart rate is going up, down, or all around. If you want to see problems coming early for every patient you have, remember that for every number they generate, you must know where that number falls into that patient's continuum or you will miss the signs of compensation every single time.

Numbers standing alone are meaningless, misleading, and may even be ticking time bombs. You have no idea if the patient is better or worse if you are not looking at trends.. Maybe your post-op patient with the 110 heart rate came out of surgery with a heart rate of 130; the next day it was 120, and today it is 110. What is happening with this patient? That's right, he's getting better.

After a crisis, if you go back into the patient's chart, clues of the coming catastrophe can be clearly seen in the heart rate starting to climb, respiratory rate starting to climb, and urine output less than before. But that is hindsight. Anyone can see things in hindsight. The real skill is in seeing it coming in real time and your clue in this post-op patient is heart rate starting to climb. Heart rate starting to climb is your first sign from patients who are bleeding, getting fluid overloaded, hypoxic, or infected.

Hemodynamic Principals, Shock, and Heart Failure

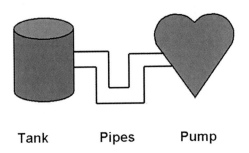

Tank   Pipes   Pump

Figure 4-3. Tank, Pipes, Pump

Your cardiovascular system is made of your tank, your pipes, and your pump. The tank is the blood volume, the pipes are the blood vessels, and the pump is your heart.

You may hear people say, "*He's two quarts low. He's running on empty. We need to top off his tank.*" They are talking about blood volume. The type of shock you get when your tank is empty is called *hypovolemic*, and it doesn't matter how you got there. I could have given you too much Lasix or you could have grabbed the stop sign. Hypovolemic is *hypovolemic*.

The pipes are the blood vessels – how dilated or constricted they are. It is called the *systemic vascular resistance*, or *pulmonary vascular resistance* if you are in the lungs. There are three types of shock that have to do with the pipes being too big. They are 1) *septic* – massive vasodilatation from endotoxins, 2) *anaphylactic* – massive vasodilatation from an allergic reaction, and 3) *neurogenic* – seen in patients with spinal cord injuries.

The pump in the system is the heart. Contractility of the heart is impacted by blood flow, availability of oxygen to make ATP to form actin – myosin bridges, and whether there was an action potential asking the heart to squeeze. Blood must flow through the heart to drop off the good stuff and pick up to carry away the bad stuff. We will look at what pushes the blood through the coronary arteries in just a minute.

What do you call pump failure? *Cardiogenic* shock. These

three forms of shock require different treatments. What is the treatment for the patient in hypovolemic shock? Fluids. If the tank is empty, fill it up. For the patient with a distributive shock, when the pipes got bigger, the inner lumen of the vessels increased, and the fluid level in the tank dropped. We have the same volume in a greater area. Current therapy for the patient with a distributive shock is to make sure the tank is filled back up before ever adding a vasoconstrictor – the reason being that when you tighten down on someone's pipes, it greatly increases the workload of the heart, and you don't want to do that unless you absolutely have to. You can tell if your patient's tank is full using the central venous pressure (CVP) or their pulmonary artery pressure if you have the right equipment.

For the patient in hypovolemic shock, you have fluid running lickety-split. For the patient in one of the distributive shocks, you have fluid going lickety-split and possibly a vasoconstrictor. But what happens to the patient in cardiogenic shock if you give him four liters of normal saline? You just killed him, didn't you? Which begs the question, why is the patient in cardiogenic shock so different from patients with other forms of shock?

Coronary Artery Blood Flow

The coronary arteries take off out of the cusps of the aortic valve, course across the top of the heart (where they can easily be bypassed by a cardiac surgeon) but then they turn and dive into the myocardium. When they do this, they become very easily compressed. The myocardium gets its blood supply during diastole. So the force shoving the blood down the coronary arteries is the diastolic blood pressure.

A patient called me into her room and complained of a 5/10 of her usual and accustomed chest pain. She requested a NTG tablet. Since I was a wonderful nurse, I got her blood pressure before giving it to her. She had a pressure of 110/60. Can this patient have a NTG tablet? What is the rule? Systolic blood pressure must be greater than 100 mmHg. So, I gave her the NTG tablet and within seconds we had a pressure of 70/40. A diastolic pressure of 40 mmHg was insufficient to perfuse her coronary arteries and she went right into cardiogenic shock. (I went right behind her.) She turned that lovely grey-green color we all hate to see in our patients, and she was waving good-bye.

When it was all over and she was stable again, I went back into her chart trying to figure out what I had done wrong. I found that her normal blood pressure was 190/100. This was in the days when we believed elderly people needed high blood pressures to perfuse their stenotic carotid arteries. We gave up on that and started doing endarterectomies. This is the first time I ever heard the term *relative* shock. I thought shock was defined by a systolic blood pressure of less than100 mmHg. In those days it was. Now it more like a systolic pressure of 90 or maybe 80 depending on the patient. It is also any time there has been more than a 40 point systolic drop, and my patient had just had an 80 point drop in her systolic pressure. She was in shock before I ever gave her the nitroglycerine tablet, and by giving it to her, I almost killed her.

The mistake I made was that I took emergency numbers and compared them to the norms I learned in school. Don't ever do that. When taking emergency numbers on a patient, always go back and compare those numbers to the *patient's* normal numbers, not to some normal in your head that you learned in school. Our patients are notorious for coming into the hospital having not read the book describing normal numbers, normal behavior, etc. Always compare the emergency numbers to the patient's normal numbers or you have a set up for making big mistakes.

As I found out with this patient, you need to keep in mind three things: relative shock, relative bradycardia, and relative anemia. In fact, there is actually relative *everything* because it always depends on *what is normal for this patient*.

Acute Congestive Heart Failure

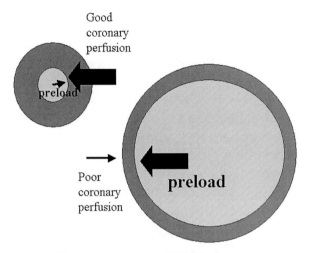

Figure 4-4. Acute CHF Diagram

If you put a whole lot of blood into the heart, it stretches the walls way out and they become thinner. The coronary arteries still course across the top of the heart, but when they turn and dive into the myocardium, they have a heck of a time getting any blood into the muscle. The volume of blood in the heart and the pressure it puts on the walls is called the *preload*. The blood is forced down the coronary arteries by the diastolic blood pressure, but its flow is opposed by the volume of blood in the ventricle (chamber) and the pressure it creates – the *preload*.

Are you having trouble understanding the concepts surrounding the preload and afterload? So did I; I don't know how many years I spent trying to understand the concepts of preload and afterload until someone told me that the pressures are *pre-* and *after-* the aortic valve. That insight went a long way in helping me understand these concepts.

The more volume in the heart, the less able you are to perfuse the myocardium. This fluid overload state is called *congestive heart failure*. The problem in CHF is that there is too much blood in the heart; diastolic pressure driving coronary artery blood flow is compromised, so you can't deliver oxygen to the cells for them to make ATP and run their action potentials and contract. The result is a poor squeeze in the heart with resultant pulmonary edema and hypoxia. This patient can have a lethal dysrhythmia and die.

To treat this patient with an acute CHF, we must unload the volume and move the patient to a lesser preload so that more flow can come down the coronary arteries, which should prevent death by lethal dysrhythmia. To help ourselves in this endeavor, we will use oxygen, Lasix, digitalis, NTG, and morphine. This is the patient with an acute CHF, not a chronic one, so we won't use beta blockers or ACE inhibitors.

The first thing on our list is oxygen.

I went down to the ER one day to help out (I'm a CNS) because they were having "the day from Hell." There were two cardiac arrests happening simultaneously and a patient having an acute MI. The novice nurse was with the MI patient, so I went to see if I could help her. I noticed that the patient didn't have any oxygen going. I asked the novice if she would like me to put some O2 on her patient. She replied that he didn't need it since his O2 saturation was 97%.

What had she missed? Where do you want this oxygen? In his finger tip or in the ischemic area of his heart? Patients having cardiac events always get oxygen! If the patient is a CO2 retaining COPDer, they, more than anyone else, will need the extra oxygen to make it through the crisis and repolarize his action potential. You just don't put it on and leave it on. You make him better and then bring down the oxygen.

I put oxygen on the patient having the MI. There was now little Os getting into the heart muscle. The patient used this oxygen to make ATP to run his action potential so he didn't die of a lethal dysrhythmia, and he squeezed with it. Increased contractility equals increased stroke volume. Improved emptying drops the preload, thereby increasing flow down the coronary arteries, which increases the chances of having a living patient.

Oxygen is an extremely benign thing to do to someone in the short term. If you had a CO2 retaining COPDer, you might make his PCO2 go up. Might. The beauty of oxygen is that you can always take it off. But remember, you squeeze with oxygen and you run your action potential with it. It is nice to have around for that reason.

Next on our list is Lasix. Lasix helps this patient drop his preload through the elimination of extra fluid. If it is in the toilet, it's not available to come back into the heart, and the dropped preload allows more flow down the coronary arteries. Remember, all things can also go too far and have negative consequences. You don't want to unload your patient too much, or you drop the blood pressure that forces the blood down the coronary arteries, and you still get poor myocardial perfusion. All things within moderation, please.

Digitalis helps the patient to increase myocardial contractility and thereby squeeze better and empty better. Digitalis also lowers the heart rate. Nothing consumes oxygen in the heart the way heart rate does. It gets about 85% of the available oxygen. Therefore, dropping someone's heart rate (within reason) saves oxygen that can be used to run the action potential and squeeze with.

In the ICU, you may see the doctor use other drugs that increase contractility, such as a Milrinone drip, or decrease heart rate, such as a beta blocker, but the effect is the same: increase contractility and decrease oxygen consumption. If you can't get more oxygen into the myocardium, the next best thing is to decrease consumption so there is some left over for contractility and running the action potential.

If you give someone a nitroglycerine tablet, it causes his peripheral blood vessels to dilate and lowers his blood pressure. Blood pressure is a large component of afterload. Afterload is the amount of pressure the chamber needs to generate in order to open the valve and empty its contents.

Therefore, the first part of afterload to consider is the quality of the valve in question. If the valve leaflets are just little tissue paper things that easily lay back against the aorta – the way they should – it doesn't take much energy to move them. But if the valve leaflets are stuck together and you have to push pretty hard to open them, or if you have a tight stenotic opening that you are trying to cram all the blood thorough, that will require even more energy, and the pressure measured as afterload goes up, decreasing emptying.

Once you get the valve open, blood pressure is a very large component of afterload, but remember to also consider the consistency of the blood and compliance of the blood vessels. It is harder to shove around sludge then it is to shove around fruit punch. Your patient's hematocrit is a part of their afterload as is the compliance of the blood vessels. If the vessels are young and healthy, they easily bulge out with each bolus of blood. Not much energy is required. But if you have tough, old stenotic blood vessels, or if you have a vasoconstrictor on the outside of the blood vessels, it will increase the workload for the heart. And the afterload goes up.

Our next treatment for the acute CHF patient is morphine. In this instance, morphine is not for pain; it is there to decrease the circulating catecholamines. The catecholamines are the neurotransmitters for the sympathetic nervous system that make your heart rate and blood pressure go up. If the heart rate and blood pressure don't go up, you save oxygen that can be used to run the action potential and squeeze with.

Decreasing circulating catecholamines can be done with a Valium tablet. The problem is that the Valium takes forever to get into the bloodstream and forever to get back out. You want something that is fast-acting and quickly metabolized if you decide that you no longer want it around. Morphine fits that bill. It is also a big time vasodilator, which you need to keep in mind. Some doctors are switching to Dilaudid or Fentanyl, feeling that either of these drugs has fewer side effects. You should always do what works best for this particular patient.

BNP (Natrecor) is a new treatment on the market for congestive heart failure. It is both a treatment and a diagnostic tool. Sometimes it is difficult to determine whether a patient is having an MI or is in congestive heart failure, and you need to know as treatments vary. Measuring serum BNP levels can tell you. The numbers are elevated in patients with CHF. If you have CHF, the clinician can infuse BNP into the patient as a vasodilator and preload reducer.

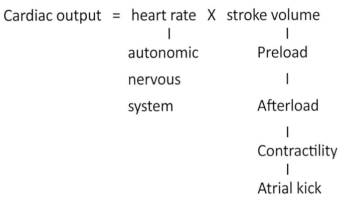

Cardiac output is heart rate times stroke volume. Heart rate is a factor of sympathetic/parasympathetic innervation into the SA node and the four factors of pH, electrolytes, glucose and oxygen. Stroke volume has several components. The first is preload. You can't get out what you didn't put in. Afterload is resistance to flow -- the higher it is, the less well the heart empties. Contractility – how hard did you squeeze, and did you get your atrial kick – signified by one p in front of every QRS. These are the components of stroke volume.

If you give someone a cardiac medication, you do it to improve their cardiac output by manipulating any of the above factors. By the same token, if your patient has a problem in any of these areas, it negatively affects cardiac output and you need to get it fixed.

Symptoms of Left and Right Heart Failure

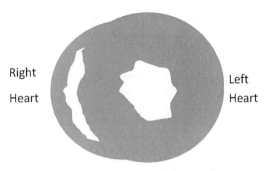

Right
Heart
Left
Heart

Figure 4-5. Heart with L and R

We are forever showing students diagrams of the cardiovascular system that make you think that the right heart looks the same as the left heart. They don't look anything like each other. If you took a heart (turkey and beef are good, chicken a little hard to see, and human not recommended), cut it in half, and turned it on its side, in the center you would see an inconstant inner lumen of the left ventricle and a large muscle mass around it. To the outside of the large muscle mass, there is a slit with a thin muscle mass around it. This is the right ventricle. The right ventricle literally wraps around the left ventricle. They don't look anything like each other while having the same volumes. But we teachers are forever showing you diagrams that make you think they do.

The left and right ventricles are totally separate entities. You could have one behind your knee and one behind your ear and it would work out fine. The problem is that you need them to beat in synchrony and if you put them up against each other and let them share a conduction system, your synchronization problem is solved.

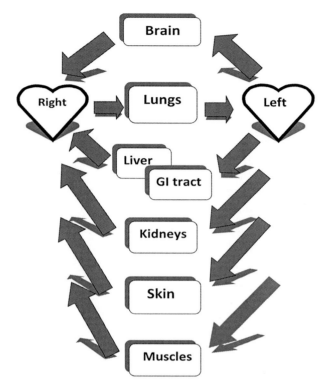

Figure 4-6. Cardiovascular Circuit

Next, we are going to look at right and left heart failure. I know it is possible to ruin your right heart with your left heart, and vice versa, and that people do it all the time – it is called biventricular failure. But, for the purposes of this teaching example, we will look at pure right and pure left heart failure. The deoxygenated blood leaves the right heart and goes to the lungs where the RBCs once again saturate it to the best of their ability with oxygen. The blood then goes to the left ventricle, where it is pumped out into the systemic circulation, where the oxygen and other good things are delivered to the cells. The deoxygenated blood then comes back into the right heart, where it is pumped into the lungs, and the journey begins again.

Around and around it goes in a clockwise – and only clockwise – fashion, unless you have holes in places where they don't belong. (We aren't going to talk about those patients.)

Because the blood moves only in a clockwise fashion, should you obstruct the blood flow anywhere in the system, you will see the pressure begin to back up downstream from the trouble.

Right Heart Failure

We will begin first with right heart failure. There are numerous things that can cause your right heart to fail. You can infarct it, get a myopathy, or one very efficient way to make it fail is for the pressure in the lungs to go up. The thin-walled right ventricle cannot push against high pressures, and it fails. *Cor pulmonale* is right heart failure secondary to *pulmonary hypertension*. For whatever reason, we now have right heart failure.

Because the blood cannot flow smoothly through the right heart, pressure begins to back up downstream. One of the first places you see a problem is in the liver. The liver becomes engorged and enlarges. We say the liver drops because it can be easily felt down in the abdomen. The liver is responsible for the metabolism of fats, carbohydrates, and protein. It makes precursors to hormones, clotting factors, and is a huge filter. None of this is going to work well when it is engorged.

The guts also become engorged as the walls swell from the increased pressure. Nutrition is crucial for keeping your patients alive, but they are supposed to absorb the nutrients through the microvillus in the small intestine, and these are swollen closed. Right heart failure patients have lots of digestive and nutrition problems.

Urine is made in the kidneys by a pure pressure-driven system. If the pressure distal to the kidney goes up, the amount of urine being made goes down. Besides urine production, the kidneys are responsible for balancing pH, electrolytes, fluid, and removing waste products. All are things that, if not done right, can make you dead. Kidney function is very important to health and well being.

The pressure also backs up into the skin, causing these patients to have edematous extremities. Blood flows through the muscles dropping off oxygen to make ATP to exercise with. If the pressure distal goes up, flow goes down, and the exercise capacity drops off.

The brain is also trying to send blood back into the right heart, and it also becomes edematous and you get a change in mentation. Everything in life occurs along a continuum. You can have so much of whatever it is that you just died from it, or so little of it we can hardly tell you have it. When you look at the change in mentation continuum, at one end is obtunded and unresponsive to pain. At the other end of the continuum the signs may be so subtle you can hardly perceive them.

Mild 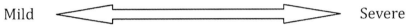 Severe

Continuum

It can be as subtle as a change in personality. If you have a patient who has been a sweetheart who is now a bear, take a look at his I&O. Nine times out of ten, you have a patient who is getting fluid overloaded. For women, once a month the world goes out of whack – we stay the same, but the world gets weird. We think what happens is that women retain a lot of fluid, giving them a touch of cerebral edema, and irritability is a sign of the cerebral edema. If you have a patient who appears suddenly irritable check the patient's I&O before getting involved in a confrontation.

Other things that are early signs of change in mentation are the patient who you only had to tell once yesterday, but have had to tell him twice today. Or maybe you are in the patient's room walking around and he isn't paying any attention to you. If someone was walking around your bedroom, would you be paying attention? Of course you would. Especially if that person is known to carry enema tubes and needles in her hands, you should be paying close attention! If you speak to a patient, he may answer appropriately, and then just drift away. This could be another early sign of change in mentation.

It is possible to ruin the left heart with the right heart and vice versa; it is called biventricular failure. But for the purposes of this explanation, let's continue to discuss only pure right and pure left heart failure.

You have a patient with a pure right heart failure. Can you hear crackles in the lungs? No? Why not? Because, the lungs are not downstream from the right heart. Can you hear crackles in the lungs of patients with a pure left heart failure? You bet, because the lungs are now downstream.

There are two kinds of heart failure patients. There are the ones to whom you give one cc too much fluid and they just crash and burn. These are actually the easy ones to take care of because their problems are obvious. The hard ones to care for are the ones with better compensatory mechanisms, because they will compensate and keep compensating, and then crash and burn in the middle of the night when you least expect it.

I did a study at our hospital of the second group of patients – the ones who got so fluid overloaded without anyone noticing that they ended up in the intensive care unit. When I went back into these patients' charts, I could tell you what shift the patient went into failure on. Not what day, but what shift they went into heart failure on. *"That is swell,"* you say, *"but that is hindsight and anyone can figure something out in hindsight."* Yes, the real problem is doing it in real time. But, you have to ask yourself, *"What was I looking for?"* I knew to look for the signs of compensation in the body, or what I like to call *the subclinical signs of impending doom* – which are, again, the heart rate and respiratory rate go up and the urine output is less than it had been before.

Let's stay in the lungs and see why the respiratory rate starts to climb. If someone is going into heart failure, the first thing he does before dumping a lot of fluid into the alveolar space where it can be heard as crackles, the first thing he does is to swell up his intersticium – the space between the cells. This increases the distance oxygen has to diffuse to make it to the capillary and the patient becomes hypoxic. The body depends on oxygen to make its only source of energy. If the amount of oxygen in the circulatory system is dropping off, the first thing the body does to compensate is to increase the respiratory rate.

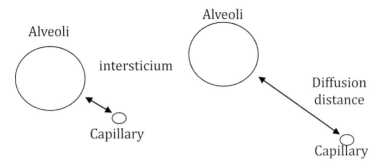

The younger and healthier the patient is, the longer they will be able to compensate by raising the respiratory rate. When compensation fails, then you get all the symptoms we learned in school – the patients say they feel short of breath, junk in the lungs, and the numbers drop off; but the first thing the patient does is to increase his respiratory rate. The patient was breathing 12 times a minute yesterday and had an O2 saturation of 97. The patient is breathing 20 times a minute today and has an O2 saturation of 97%. Is there a change? Would your nurse's aide have picked up on it? This is the second sign of compensation: the patient is working harder to stay in exactly the same place.

Let's move into the heart and see why the heart rate starts to climb in the patients going into heart failure. Cardiac output = heart rate X stroke volume. This makes heart rate a very interesting vital sign. Things that make the heart rate go up and down include hypoxia, fever, exercise, change in stroke volume because of overload or underload, etc. But, let's say the patient isn't bleeding out, or hypoxic, septic, or jumping up and down on the bed, but the heart rate is going up and down. What you are looking at are changes in myocardial contractility. If all the other factors are stable, heart rate is a direct look into the patient's heart at how well it is contracting.

In our patient with left heart ischemia from whatever reason (myopathy, infarction, too high a preload, etc.), the heart is squeezing less well and the heart rate will pick up in an attempt to keep the cardiac output adequate to meet the body's metabolic needs. The purpose of the left heart is to pump the oxygenated blood through the systemic circulation and out to the cells. In order to get the blood to the body's cells, the perfusion pressure must stay high enough, but we have poor squeeze and the perfusion pressures have dropped off. In order to compensate for the lower pressure, the body will vasoconstrict throughout the cardiovascular circuit.

Once the blood vessels are vasoconstricted, blood pressure is no longer a good indicator of how the patent is doing. If the blood pressure is low, indeed you do have a problem, but don't be fooled into thinking everything is OK because the blood pressure is normal or high. If you have a vasoconstricted patient, blood pressure may not be a good indicator of how the patient is doing, but heart rate is. Heart rate is a direct look into the patient's heart at how well it is squeezing (contractility). If the heart is squeezing well, stroke volume goes up. To compensate for the increased volume, heart rate goes down. Squeeze less well, heart rate goes up; squeeze better, heart rate goes down to maintain the same cardiac output.

So, the patient in left heart failure is frequently vasoconstricted throughout the body. Vasoconstrict into the brain and you get the same change of mentation anywhere along the continuum of mild to obtunded. Vasoconstrict into the liver and it doesn't work any better than it did all engorged and it can be infarcted. Vasoconstrict into the guts and you can have very serious problems.

Inside our digestive system, we have some very caustic substances – hydrochloric acid, pancreatic enzymes – things there to help us digest our food. These are non-selective digesters. They would be happy to digest us at the same time. To protect us from this unfortunate (and painful) event, we have a wonderful gastric mucosa. It must be repaired constantly, using the food we eat, that comes via the circulatory system, and using ATP as an energy source. If there is decreased blood flow into the gut, we don't repair the mucosa as well as we should. It is also possible to infarct and make ulcers.

Our digestive system is home to three to four hundred species of bacteria. They are our friends. We want them there. But, we want them there under our conditions. One of those conditions is that the colony counts must stay down. To keep the colony counts down, every day or so we deposit multitudes of them into the toilet and flush them away. This requires peristalsis, which requires muscle contraction, which requires blood flow, ATP, etc., etc. Decreased blood flow into the gut decreases peristalsis, which allows the bacteria live long lives, reproduce constantly, and pump all kinds of toxins into the patient making them feel awful. Left heart failure patients have lots of GI distress.

Vasoconstrict into the kidneys and urinary output starts to drop off anywhere on the continuum of mild to completely shut down. In our study patients, none of them had abnormally low urine outputs before their great crash. Most of them had more than 500 cc urine out a shift, which would send off no warnings unless you are looking at trends. With the same or greater intake, every shift the urine output was less than the shift before is a sign of vasoconstriction of the renal artery. At the time of these patients' crises, they all stopped making urine, but early on, urine output was just less than it had been before.

Vasoconstrict into the skin and we will see the cold, clammy, diaphoretic skin. We now know that diaphoresis is a very ominous sign. It is a sympathetic response that uses a parasympathetic neurotransmitter. That's nice, but why should you care? Because any patient who is diaphoretic is maximally sympathetically stimulated. They are using everything they have to keep those numbers right where they are. One more little bitty *anything* and they crash and burn. A diaphoretic patient is a crisis waiting to happen.

If you vasoconstrict into the muscles, less oxygen is delivered, less ATP made, and exercise capacity will go down.
What we have been looking at are the non-invasive signs of poor cardiac output. These are things you can see in the patient without having to send them to the diagnostic center and without having a million dollar machine come to the bedside. These signs are:

1. A change in mentation, anywhere along the continuum
2. Respiratory distress, anywhere along the continuum
3. The heart rate is up
4. The liver is engorged
5. GI problems have increased
6. Urine output has dropped off
7. The skin is edematous and/or cold, clammy, and diaphoretic, and
8. Exercise capacity has decreased.

If you are working with a patient in an acute situation, and you want to know how good a job you are doing of oxygenating and perfusing the patient's cells, I think there are three good indicators. They don't come in any order; they frequently come all at once. They are: 1) a change in mentation, because neurons are so sensitive to hypoxia; 2) rate of ectopy (irregular heartbeats) because the action potential is so sensitive to hypoxia, and 3) diaphoresis because it shows maximal sympathetic stimulation. Any of these symptoms getting better – nice work! Any of them getting worse – work harder! If the patient flutters his eyes open and looks at you – good job! If he rolls his eyes back in his head – work harder!

In the long run, if you want to know how a patient is doing, the improvement can be measured in exercise capacity. If a patient has come to you to get better, they should be better every single day and it can be seen as an improvement in exercise capacity. How do you know if a patient is increasing his exercise capacity? You measure it, and make sure all the people in your work area are using the same yardstick – you have to have concrete markers that all staff recognize. In one hospital, they have 25 foot markers on the wall, so they can say the patient went 25 feet, 100 feet, 350 feet. Other units may use parts of a loop of their work area, whatever, as long as everyone agrees on the form of measurement so you know that everyone is talking the same language.

What do you mean when you say the patient ambulated well? What I mean is that the patient had no signs of poor cardiac output the whole time he was being ambulated. That is a nurse's decision to make, not a nurse's aide's. In an ideal situation, you and the aide would ambulate the patient, but we seldom get ideal. The least I want you to settle for is to watch it happen. Tell the aide that when she is going to ambulate the patient, she should let you know. Then make sure to watch it happen, because whether or not the patient ambulated well is *your* decision.

If a patient needs oxygen to lie in bed, do they need oxygen to walk down the hall? *Yes!* Nurse's aides do not understand this. In their two weeks of nursing school, ATP formation and action potentials never came up once They don't know the link between oxygen and heartbeat. You do. So if the patient needs oxygen to lie passively in bed, he will need oxygen to walk down the hall. If you are going to increase someone's exercise or stress level (like going to the diagnostic center), the patient needs their prescribed oxygen, not less! If you deny the patient his oxygen, your walk will turn into a drag. There will be two or more of you dragging the hypoxic patient back to bed!

We are forever assigning knowledge to nurse's aides that they do not have. Because they do their chores well, we think they understand the reason behind the action, but they often don't. They are simply repeating actions without understanding underlying cause or treatment goals. It is the *nurse* who possesses this knowledge. It is the *nurse* who needs to guide the aide; the nurse who understands the why. Keep control.

Time for a quick quiz.

> *What are the things that make you heart rate go up?*
> Stroke volume falling because you are under or over loaded
> Hypoxia
> Fever
> Sympathetic stimulation (pain, fear, anxiety)
> Exercise
> Drugs
>
> *What are things that make your respiratory rate go up?*
> Hypoxia
> Compensation for metabolic acidosis
> Exercise
> Sympathetic Stimulation
> Psychological Factors

Number one is hypoxia! Always confirm that the patient is not hypoxic before dragging out the Haldol. Hypoxia makes you very anxious and if the people around you are saying stupid things like, "*Slow your breathing down,*" or "*Just relax,*" it is pretty easy to come unglued because you know you are having a life-threatening event and you can't get anyone to believe you.

Metabolic acidosis will increase the respiratory rate as the patient tries to compensate for his lactic acidosis by hyperventilating and "blowing off" CO_2. The body tries to compensate for the high lactic acid content by getting rid of another acid present, like CO_2, and thereby bring the pH back to normal. If you ever have a patient breathing too fast for no apparent respiratory reason, ask yourself whether or not it might be compensation for lactic acidosis.

I was asked to see a patient in the diagnostic center who had just had his bilateral nephrostomy tubes replaced. The radiology tech had called and said, "I don't know what is wrong with him. He just doesn't look right. Would you come see him?" I told him I would be right there. When I arrived, the patient was sitting on the gurney. His blood pressure and heart rate were slightly elevated and he was somewhat flushed, but placing nephrostomy tubes is hard, painful work. He was also breathing deep and fast. Being the excellent nurse that I am, I felt this was something that needed to be followed up on. I whipped out my stethoscope, placed it on his chest, and I clearly heard normal breath sounds throughout both lungs. I asked him if he was short of breath and he said, "*No.*" I said, "*Why are you breathing so fast?*" and he said, "*I don't know.*" Within 30 minutes he was in the ICU, on a ventilator in septic shock. The increased respirations were his compensation for the lactic acidosis being caused by his incipient sepsis. He must have had a pocket of some very virulent organisms left over from another set of tubes, and when they placed these tubes, they must have gone right through it, showering the organism throughout his body for him to be that sick, that fast. If you ever have a patient breathing too fast for no apparent respiratory reason, wonder to yourself whether or not it might be compensation for a metabolic acidosis – and in our work environment, sepsis is the most likely candidate.

Other things that make your respiratory rate go up are exercise and sympathetic stimulation. Another cause for an increase in respiration is anxiety. I have a very hard time with the psychological diagnosis being given because the most likely recipients are women. Men have diseases, women have hysteria. Hysteria, uterus, hysterectomy. See the connection. For years it was felt that men could *not* be hysterical, only women. Of course, the women might have become hysterical when they couldn't get the doctor to understand there was something wrong with them that could not be fixed with a hysterectomy.

Key Components to Chapter 4

1. Things that happen during diastole are: filling, repolarization, and coronary perfusion.
2. Blood flows in the cardiac circuit from high pressure to low pressure, but the low pressure draws blood to it.
3. The cardiac cycle includes passive and active (atrial kick) filling and systole. You need an intact column of fluid, distensible heart and pressure in just the right places.
4. CO = HR X SV. HR is driven by autonomic nervous system stimulation, stroke volume, fever, and metabolic factors. SV is composed of preload (volume in the heart), afterload (resistance to flow), contractility (how hard did you squeeze, and did you have one p in front of each QRS (atrial kick).
5. Before the body becomes ill, it tries to compensate for the problem. Signs of compensation are heart rate and respiratory rates starting to climb and urine output less than it had been before.
6. Signs of heart failure include changes in mentation anywhere on the continuum, heart rate starting to climb, respiratory distress anywhere on the continuum, increase in GI problems, liver is down, urine output less than it had been with the same or greater intake, peripheral edema/pale, cold, clammy, or diaphoretic skin, and a decrease in exercise capacity.
7. Goals of the treatment of heart failure are:
   a. Prevent overload using ACE and β blockers
   b. Cure overload using drugs that decrease preload and afterload, increase contractility, and decrease the workload of the heart
   c. Increase coronary artery perfusion and increase oxygen delivery to the myocardial cells so the patient can make ATP, use it to run his action potential, squeeze his heart, and go on to live another day.

Chapter 5
Acute Respiratory Distress

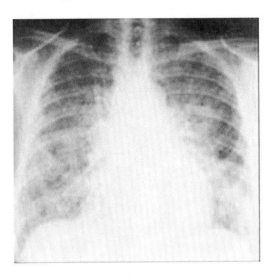

Figure 5-1. Chest X-ray ARDS

Acute Respiratory Distress Syndrome (ARDS) is a catastrophic event that can lead to a disastrous outcome. Whether your patient will survive depends on the patent's resources going into the event, the severity of the causative agent, and whether or not the event has been curtailed. Overriding these three factors is how long things went undetected and untreated. A key to surviving ARDS is early detection and treatment, frequently requiring an ICU bed and a ventilator.

Before we can delve into what goes wrong in ARDS, we need to study the inflammatory process. When people speak of the response to injury, they are talking about inflammation. The body uses the inflammatory process to clean up debris, heal wounds, make scars, and re-establish functioning.

Inflammation, like everything else, appears on a continuum. It's possible to have too much or too little. Let's take a look at the middle ground.

Everything you do physiologically – the beating of your heart, the breathing of your lungs, the digesting of your food, the macro vasculature – is about the exchange that takes place between the micro-capillaries and their adjoining cells. They drop off the good stuff, then pick up the bad stuff and carry it away. A great deal of the immune system is contained in the capillaries, but the problem is frequently outside the capillaries in the area around the cells. There needs to be a method for getting the white blood cell (WBC) in the circulation to come out of the blood vessel to attack the problem.

At this point, the micro-capillary walls are the thickness of one-cell. Between each cell in the wall are slit pores that can be opened and closed on command. When the slit pore is opened, the white cell comes out,and the pore closes back up again. When the pores are opened, the first thing that happens is that plasma pours out and will continue to pour out until it closes up.

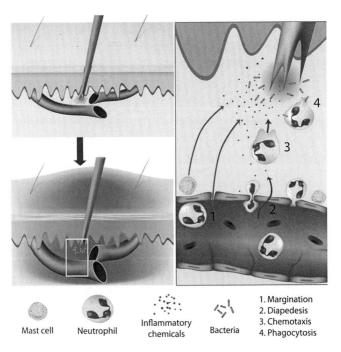

| | | Inflammatory chemicals | Bacteria | 1. Margination
2. Diapedesis
3. Chemotaxis
4. Phagocytosis |
| Mast cell | Neutrophil | | | |

Figure 5-2. Inflammation

Because red blood cells (RBC) are much smaller than WBC, do you suppose when the slits are opened wide enough to let out WBC that some RBCs might escape also? (Sure they do.)

Imagine that your skin was punctured by a thorn. When the thorn went through the skin, it damaged cells and brought in bacteria. The damaged cells need to be removed, the bacteria eliminated, and the skin repaired. It is the inflammatory process that will do this for us.

The general in this battle against the invaders is a roving T cell. There are patrols of B cells out looking for invaders; if they spot one, they deliver the information to the T cell and prepare for battle by multiplying like crazy. The T cell needs to call for its warriors – the white cells in the bloodstream. The vast majority of the white cells in your body are not floating around where you can count them with a CBC, they are marginated – clinging to the walls of the blood vessel. This is how you can have a normal white count one day and 20,000 the next. You didn't make the white cells overnight; they were already there waiting to be called, kind of like in suspended animation – which is a really neat way to keep your warriors until you need them.

The T cell secretes a series of chemical mediators to make the inflammatory process happen – the mediators make things happen while the T cell makes inflammation happen. One of the first mediators secreted is a signal to the blood vessel to vasodilate – you want more blood with more white cells to mount the attack. The T cell then sends a signal to the marginated white cells and tells them to demarginate and get ready to go. If all they did was drop off the wall, they would be washed away in the circulation, but they actually get kind of sticky and stay wherever the need is.

Now, this is all really nice, but it is happening inside the blood vessel and our problem is outside the blood vessel. Luckily, our blood vessels are not lead pipes; they have those slit pores that can be opened up. Chemical mediators from the T cell tell the capillary to increase its permeability, which opens the pores and lets the white cells migrate out. At this point, the capillary pores are open and the white cells are out, but they don't know where to go.

However, the T cell has laid down a chemotaxic smell trail; the white cells *smell* their way up to the problem. When they get there, they begin to secrete proteases that destroy proteins so they can clean up the debris and begin to phagocytize the bacteria. They know what to get, because the T cell and the complementary system mark things, putting tags on the bad guys which say, "Get this one, not that one." This is how your body knows what is you and what isn't you – host verses graft.

This is the inflammatory process. The physical signs of inflammation reflect the pathophysiology going on. The redness and heat come from vasodilation, the swelling from increased capillary permeability, and the exudate from the white cell attack on the bacteria. Pain is generated by pressure on the nerves from the swelling and by direct irritation of the nerves by chemical mediators, and is a way of getting the individual's attention to the problem so that maybe he will pluck the thorn out and aid the healing process.

Inflammation is a delightful process that is meant to be localized. If you take it and spread it throughout your entire body it is called Systemic Inflammatory Response Syndrome (SIRS) and is a very bad idea. We had never had a patient with SIRS, or its respiratory component ARDS, until we invented the ventilator, because before there were ventilators, they would have died and we would never have seen it. As we now have ventilators, we have a way of keeping people alive past the point where – in the past – they would have died, and we can see all kinds of normal compensatory mechanism going amok in the patient's body.

The first time we noticed ARDS was during the Viet Nam War. It was the first time we had ventilators on a large number of people in one area. Before the war, a hospital might have a ventilator or two, but no one had a lot of them. But in the Viet Nam War, there were a lot of healthy people who suffered severe traumas and would have died, but were placed on ventilators. The patient tended to do OK for a few days, then might all of a sudden get a severe hypoxia, a white out on his chest x-ray, and die despite the most heroic efforts of the medical staff. We originally called it

Da Nang lung, shock lung, wet lung, or white lung. Years later, we called it adult respiratory distress syndrome. Even later, we called it acute lung injury and acute respiratory distress syndrome.

We had also noticed that these patients tended to have cascading organ failure occur with the respiratory failure. Originally, we had said that was most unfortunate, but it had just happened. Years later, we determined that the organ failure and respiratory failure were of common origin – SIRS. ARDS is the respiratory component to SIRS, disseminated intervascular coagulopathy (DIC) is the hematological component, acute renal failure (ARF) is the renal component, liver failure (LF) in all its forms is the hepatic component, and having low blood pressure is the cardiovascular component. It hits the body all at once; you just most often see it in the lungs first.

The different components of SIRS are all tied together, so that if you were to get one, you are at risk for all the others. For example, let's suppose that you are a fireman who inhales smoke at a fire, then gets ARDS.

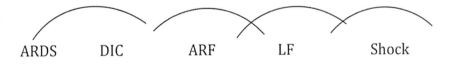

ARDS   DIC   ARF   LF   Shock

Now that you have ARDS, you are at risk for renal failure, DIC, liver failure, and cardiovascular collapse. Patients having any one of the component parts of SIRS are at risk for all the entities involved in SIRS, and having been in shock places patients at risk for liver failure, renal failure, DIC, etc. All of the components have multiple entry points, but once you have one you are at risk for all of them.

Survival depends on early pick-up of the symptoms, so who is at risk to go into SIRS and ARDS? Anyone who has been in shock for any reason at all, including cardiac syncope patients, is at risk. Sepsis is a very popular pathway into SIRS and ARDS. Trauma patients, too; the more broken bones you have, the more likely you are to go into SIRS and ARDS. People with lung contusions – that's people with seatbelt abrasions, those who have had CPR, or who have been hit, kicked, or landed on their chests. Folks with diffuse infectious pneumonias are at high risk because their pneumonia is worse than anyone else's; SARS is one type of a diffuse infectious pneumonia. Aspiration patients: if they don't get ARDS, they can get aspiration pneumonitis and dissolve their own lung tissue – not a good trade.

Anyone who has been on heart-lung bypass is at risk. Your body never intended to have its blood sucked out of it in a plastic tube, then put back in again. It considers that an injury and sets off the response to an injury – inflammation. (This is one reason we are trying to do as much open heart surgery "off pump" as possible.) People with surface burns are at risk, and of course the bigger the burn, the greater the risk. If you survived a near-drowning and now have respiratory distress, it is frequently ARDS. Also, oxygen toxicity kills via ARDS.

Those with pancreatitis are at risk because "-itis" means inflammation. Any disease ending in "itis," if sent systemic, can result in SIRS and ARDS. (I had a patient one time that went into it due to myocarditis.) DIC patients are at risk for ARDS because DIC is the hematological component of SIRS and having one component opens you up to all of them. Patients with a fat embolus are also at risk.

These are the risk factors for going into ARDS. The severity of the symptoms, the patient's reserves, and the virility of the causative agent are the keys to determining your patient's outcome.

So, what happens in ARDS? First, you have an insult to the system setting off the response to injury. Out come the mediators, the capillaries dilate (there goes the blood pressure), oxygen radicals attack cell membranes,
proteases destroy collagen and elastin (destroying things you don't want destroyed), capillary permeability increases and fluid pours out of the capillaries – there goes what little blood pressure you had left, then the lungs eventually fill with fluid.

The causative problem in SIRS and ARDS is that the capillary permeability increases, the pores open up and they are stuck open so what fluid you give the patient does not stay contained.

The Clinical Picture of ARDS

The key to patient survival is early detection. If you are supposed to pick it up, what does it look like?

1. Severe, acute
2. Rapid onset of life threatening
3. Hypoxia
4. Impaired oxygenation refractory to O2 therapy
5. Breath sounds unremarkable
6. SOB with respiratory alkalosis
7. Tachycardia
8. Agitation

It is a severe acute onset of life-threatening hypoxia that oxygen does not make better. By severe acute onset, I don't mean that it is like blowing a pneumothorax or throwing a pulmonary embolus where the patient's condition changes in seconds, but from the time the problem starts (not the time you notice it) you only have a couple of hours until that hypoxic code. If it is three a.m. and you are thinking it's OK to wait because the doctor will be here at seven a.m. – you don't have that kind of time. You need to move faster than that.

When oxygen does not make it better, that is your first big sign that what you are dealing with is ARDS and not something else. If you ever put oxygen on a patient and do not see the PO2, or O2 saturation, respond to the increase in inspired oxygen – go directly to 100% oxygen.

With ARDS, oxygen does *not* make it better. It is a life-threatening hypoxia that administering oxygen will not rectify.

I will pause here to say that like everything else, ARDS appears on a continuum. You can have so little of it we can hardly tell you have it, or you can have so much of it you quickly die a horrible death on a ventilator with multiple organ failure. Once again, let's cover the middle ground.

The first clue we might be looking at ARDS was that oxygen does not make it better. The second clue are the patient's lung sounds. They are unremarkable for such a severe hypoxia. They are *not* clear, but they do not give you a clue to the cause of the severe hypoxia. If you had a patient who was so incredibly hypoxic when you put your stethoscope on his chest, you would expect to hear terrible things like an absence of breath sounds, or unequal sounds signifying a pneumothorax or effusions, or nasty mucus rattling around – but the breath sounds are unremarkable; not clear, but unremarkable for such an incredible hypoxia. You hear them all the way down both sides. They may be a little coarse or bronchial. Maybe a wheeze here or a crackle there, but nothing that would account for such an incredible hypoxia; here's why that is.

Just as in CHF, the patient going into ARDS will first swell up the interstitium between the alveolar wall and the capillary before dumping a lot of fluid and debris into the alveolus where it can be heard with a stethoscope. This swelling increases the distance the oxygen has to diffuse across to make it into the capillary. It also decreases the size of the alveolar space where gas exchange takes place because there is an increased diffuse distance and decrease

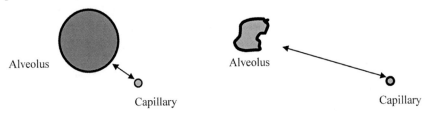

in the area for exchange to take place. The net result is a patient with a severe hypoxia but unremarkable breath sounds.

The blood gas shows a respiratory alkalosis. People with a respiratory alkalosis are frequently breathing too fast. And what is the most common cause of hyperventilation? Yes! Hypoxia! (You didn't get it right? Shame on you.) The most common cause of hyperventilation is hypoxia, but being hypoxic will make you *very* anxious.

Early on in the disease we will see the patient blowing off CO_2 as he hyperventilates from severe hypoxia. Because CO_2 exchanges across the alveolar membrane twenty times faster than oxygen does, you are very compromised before you begin to retain CO_2. Anytime a patient is retaining CO_2, that cannot be ventilated off, there has been a tremendous loss of lung functioning and the end may be near.

Keep in mind that early on, the patient blows off CO_2, but right before he dies he begins to *retain* CO_2.

The heart rate on these patients is up; what three things could be driving the patient's heart rate up? Hypoxia itself will, as the heart speeds up the delivery system for oxygen to the tissues; sympathetic stimulation causes the confused, restless, agitated, and combative response to hypoxia. How hard is the patient working to breathe?

Move on to the patient's heart. When he got so incredibly hypoxic, did his heart squeeze better or worse? (The answer should be worse.) When the capillary permeability increased and fluid poured out, what happened to stroke volume in the heart? Up or down? To compensate for this loss in cardiac output does the heart rate go up or down? Up. These are the things driving the patient's heart rate up. The heart rate going up is compensation for all the patient's problems.

What happens if the patient is taking a beta blocker when the event occurs? He isn't able to compensate. Beta blockers are wonderful drugs. They keep your patient from overcompensation; they also keep your patient from compensating in a time of stress. Be aware of beta blockers. If you think your patient may be bleeding but his heart rate isn't going up, or he is hypoxic but his heart rate isn't going up, take a look at his medication list. I bet you anything this patient is taking a beta blocker or a calcium channel blocker on board. What percentage of your patients take beta blockers? If you work with cardiac patients I would say 100%; everyone else, maybe as many as 75%. Watch out for these drugs!

And speaking of agitation, why is the patient so agitated? Because he's hypoxic. This is very easy to spot in a learning situation, but what if you are having a busy day, Mrs. Jones has just disconnected her IV again, you have to call Dr. Intimidation and tell him how you accidentally pulled out his surgical patient's J-tube while changing his gown, and you have a patient down the hall saying unkind things about you and your mother. This last patient has a particularly nasty mouth, tattoos all over him, and earrings in places you wouldn't dream of putting an earring. He is restless, and combative. What is wrong with this patient? Drug withdrawal? Maybe, but before you drag out the Haldol and leather restraints, please make sure he isn't hypoxic.

Another patient likely to have his hypoxia missed is the one with a psych or drug history. Always make sure your confused, restless, agitated, or combative patient is not hypoxic before proceeding any further.

The ARDS patient with the best chance of survival is the one who had his problem detected early. What are the two biggest clues to aid in early detection? First, oxygen doesn't make the hypoxia better and second, the patient has fairly normal breath sounds.

Treatment for this patient includes putting pressure into the patient's lungs (BiPAP, PEEP) to expand the compressed alveolar space. Putting pressure into someone's lungs requires a doctor's order and that is why early detection is so important. Until you get pressure into this patient's lungs, you are teetering on the edge of a hypoxic code.

Your job is *not* to run a good code. *Your job is to keep the code from ever happening.*

ARDS patients can present very vaguely at first. You might think you have a problem, but you aren't sure. This is an excellent time to call your Rapid Response Team (RRT), so you can get other people involved before things deteriorate into a crisis. As author I.J. Parker said in one of his novels, "the life force has withdrawn and the patient is in a state of negativity." That RRT is there to help you – *use them.*

Key Components to Chapter 5
1. Inflammation causes an increase in capillary permeability making blood pressure hard to control and flooding the lungs.
2. SIRS is a systemic disease. Its components are ARDS, DIC, ARF, hepatic failure, and shock secondary to low vascular volumes and decreased contractility of the heart muscle.
3. Early signs of ARDS are: oxygen does not make it better, and fairly normal breath sounds.
4. It is treated with pressure in the lungs via BiPAP or PEEP on a ventilator.
5. CO_2 exchanges across the membrane in the lungs twenty times faster than oxygen does. Retaining CO_2 is a very bad sign.

Chapter 6

Headaches

When the average person has a headache, chances are that it is a normal kind of headache. But our patients aren't average people. They are the sick, infirmed, and diseased; and if one of them says to us that he has a headache, chances are greater that it could be a malignant headache. Let's take a look at the differences between benign and malignant (or malevolent) headaches.

Malevolent Headache
- First headache in patient over 35 years old
- No precipitating factor or starts with exercise and doesn't stop
- Awakens patient from sleep
- Thunderclap onset
- Dull, persistent pain
- Unilateral or focal pain accompanied by fever, change in LOC, papilledema, change in neuro signs, or meningeal signs
- No response to medication
- No pediatric history of motion sickness
- No family history of headache

Did you know that there are people who have never had a headache? Did you know there are whole families of people who have never had a headache either? If someone is over 35 years old and has never had a headache but now has one, chances are it has a malevolent cause. One woman told me that no one in her family had headaches. Her mother had her first headache when she was 55 years old. It was the workup for that headache that found her polycythemia. A nurse told me she had never had a headache until she was 40 years old. It came with the stroke that she was having. So, if your patient has never had one and now has one, this is a clue that should not be ignored.

A headache that has no precipitating factor, or starts when you are exercising and doesn't resolve when you stop exercising, is not usually benign in origin. Bad headaches that awaken you from sleep or can have a thunderclap onset (sudden intense pain without gradual buildup), and dull, persistent pain that doesn't move around very much is a sign of a malevolent headache.

Unilateral or focal pain accompanied by fever, change in LOC, papilledema, change in neuro signs, or meningeal signs is a malevolent headache. If patient tells a nurse that they have a headache, very few of us stop and grab quick neuro signs, but we should. I know of a hospital that gave a family a whole bunch of money because a patient's headache did have a change in neuro signs, no nurse checked for it, and the diagnosis was missed.

Our patients are sicker than ever before, so the chance that there has been a change in neuro signs is also greater than ever before. Grab the quick neuro signs and don't forget to document them before proceeding on with treatment for the patient's headache.

Headaches that do not respond to medication are not good headaches. A pediatric history of motion sickness is related to the development of migraines in later life. If you want to know if you had a history of motion sickness as a child, try to recall family car trips. Did you get nauseated? If you did, then you do, and you are at risk to develop migraines as you get older.

Benign Headache
- Patient less than 35 years old for first one
- Precipitating factors well known
- Previous similar headaches
- Pain disappears with sleep (migraine)
- Gradual onset
- Pain described as an ice pick, jab, or squeezing
- Multifocal and/or shifting sides
- No associated systemic or neurological findings except migraine aura
- Good response to medication
- Pediatric history of motion sickness (migraine)
- Positive family history

You and I, we have the good headaches. We've had them all our lives; we know exactly what causes them. We've had thousands of them. If we can get to sleep, the headache usually goes away, although migraine sufferers can wake up with their headaches intact. It has a gradual onset, feels like the tops of our heads are blowing off, and/or it shifts from side to side in the head. Medication does make it better, we barfed in the back seat of the car, and headaches are not unknown in our families. Those are the good ones.

Pain Patterns and Headaches
- Mild onset, worsening over 1 hour then abating – migraine and tension
- Moderate at onset present on awakening, abating – arterial hypertension, sinusitis
- Worst at onset Thunderclap HA – Subarachnoid hemorrhage (persistent), Cluster HA (abating)
- Pain awakening patient at night – Cluster headache
- Pain awakening patient in the morning – neoplasm, subarachnoid bleed
- New headache, worse over time – brain abscess, meningitis
- Chronic episodic headache – Migraine, cluster, tension, or sinus HA

Headaches that start out mild, get worse, and then get better are the good ones. Headaches that are there when you wake up in the morning, but get better as you are up running around can be arterial hypertension, but are more likely sinus in origin. Sinus headaches get better as you are up and about because, the sinuses drain and the pressure/pain goes away. People who suffer from sinus headaches know that lying down flat for a long time will bring them on; being in air conditioning will do it; and having oxygen blown up your nose will occlude your sinuses in nothing flat. (And what do we do in hospitals? We bring people into air-conditioned rooms, lie them down flat, and blow oxygen up their noses!)

You don't want to throw pain medication at someone's sinus headache because you'll nauseate them. You instead want to open their sinuses up so the pain will go away. You need to know if this patient's headache is a sinus headache. But how do you find out? Ask the patient to point to the center of the headache with one finger. If the patient points to the area including the eyes and forehead it is frequently a sinus headache. If they point to anywhere else, it most likely is not a sinus headache.

Headaches that are worse at onset or have a thunder clap onset – meaning there was no gradual lead up to the pain; it was all suddenly there in full force – can be subarachnoid bleeds or cluster headaches. If you have a cerebral aneurysm ready to go, all you need do is cough, sneeze, or turn your head sharply and you can blow it wide open. I haven't turned my head sharply since I read that.

Cluster headaches are more frequently seen in men than women and are characterized by severe headaches that are episodic in nature. That is, there are periods of headaches, and periods of being headache-free. Clusters usually last two weeks to three months and are separated by at least two-week intervals of calm. They tend to occur at the same time of the day, can wake you from a deep sleep, and can be more painful than migraines. Cluster headaches appear both in the sudden onset and "wake patient from sleep at night" categories. The pain is unilateral. centered behind one eye, and often is accompanied by nausea and vomiting.

A new headache that gets worse over time requires a physician. If you have tension headaches, they all feel the same. Your sinus headaches all feel the same, as do your migraine headaches. A new type of headache is a medical emergency. Our patents usually don't differentiate between types of headaches. You have to ask the questions. "Is this your usual and accustomed headache?" "Is it in the usual strength and duration?"

> *"Is it the same or is it different"* is crucial information no matter what the patient just complained about. "Is this your usual and accustomed big toe pain? Its usual strength and duration?" Or heart pain, or any pain? Is it the same or is it different tells you if you need to go get a doctor.

If the patient says, "I have these headaches all the time," your next question for the patient needs to be what does the patient take for his headache? (Not what do you take for yours.) And if the patient says they have never had a headache like this one before, get them quickly to a doctor.

Other things that also cause headaches include problems within the eye itself or lesions of the nerves themselves, such as herpes zoster invasion, which can cause the pain of the headache to follow the affected nerve. The headache from vascular disorders can throb in time with the pulse and follow a blood vessel. Problems in the ear and mouth can also cause headaches. The headache you get from increased intracranial pressure is like no headache you have ever felt before. It has been described as more global, more intense, and just plain old different for any other headache. People who have had increased intracranial pressure know what I mean. It is a totally different kind of headache.

Inflammation, getting hit on your head, and lesions in the ear and mouth can also cause headaches. These headaches will also feel different form the patient's usual and accustomed headaches and they all require a physician.

If the patient has abnormal vision before the headache starts, don't worry about it; it is probably migraine aura. If the abnormal vision starts up after the headache begins, it could have a more sinister cause. It could be caused by an occipital vascular malformation, a problem with the posterior communicating artery, or increased intracranial pressure. Those all require a physician.

Please be aware of Horner's syndrome, which is caused by a lesion of the sympathetic nervous system causing drooping eye lid, permanent constriction of the pupil, and you don't sweat on that side of your face. It can occur with cluster headaches and be transient. If it is persistent, it can be a sign of carotid artery dissection.

Nausea and vomiting with a headache can be a sign of increased intracranial pressure, migraine, meningitis, or toxicity, but a more common cause is too much medication for the headache on an empty stomach. Always ask the patient what he has taken for his headache. Sometimes they will say, *"Well, I took about eight aspirin before I took some of that ibuprofen stuff. Then, my wife had some Tylenol with codeine left over from her surgery and I had two of them and a couple of Demerol tablets my cousin gave me yesterday."* No wonder the guy is nauseated! Before assuming increased intracranial pressure, always ask what they took for the headache.

If there is a fever with the headache, it can have an infectious or toxic origin, because you activate the response to injury to clean up debris. If the headache is accompanied by a change in LOC, papilledema, or focal neurological deficit, absolutely nothing good can be causing it and you need a doctor. Neck and back pain can be meningitis; it can also be a subarachnoid bleed.

Causes of increased intercranial pressure

- Neoplasm or tumor
- Hydrocephalus
- Pseudo tumor cerebri
- Venous stasis occlusion
- Vascular disorder
- Pressure from benign exertion

Your head is a fixed space. There is room for a certain amount of blood, gray matter, and cerebral spinal fluid. If any of those three things becomes greater in volume than it should be, or the circumference of the head becomes smaller, you get an increase in intracranial pressure. The cause of the increase in pressure can be easily seen for all of the above conditions except *pseudo* tumor cerebri. This is an idiopathic (meaning we don't know the reason it happens) intra-cranial hypertension caused because the patient doesn't reabsorb his spinal fluid the way he should. It causes a headache with a visual defect. (I found that out on Google. I can't encourage you enough to use Google day-in and day-out during your shift.)

We are all adult learners and that means we don't learn the same way we did when we were kids. When you were young, the teacher could hand you a list of something, tell you to go home, memorize it, and there would be a test on Friday. You did fine. But your memorization gene has turned off and it will never come on again. The way adults learn is by taking an event that is familiar to you and hanging a new piece of information off it; then we learn in a snap. What this means, though, is that **we need instant access to information at the time we have the question.** You may forget to look it up in your antique nursing books at home, and it's not in them anyway. It is on the Internet waiting for you.

How many times have you been asked to give a drug you can't find in the PDR or hospital formulary? I guarantee you that you'll find it on the Internet. New procedures? On the Internet. The doctor orders a lab test the lab has never heard or? **It's on the Internet. Use it, use it, use it. The best learning takes place at the time you have a need to know.**

Temporal Arteritis
- Continuous throbbing frontal HA
- Repetitive needle like pains
- Scalp tenderness
- Jaw claudication
- Temporal artery tenderness
- Diminished temporal pulses
- Visual disturbance
- Fever & elevated sed rate

Temporal arteritis is a very nasty headache. It is a continuous, constant, throbbing headache. If you give the patient narcotics it will knock him out, and when he awakens, the headache is still right there with all its intensity. This headache is caused by an inflammation of the temporal artery. If you are looking for it in the patient, you might be able to see a low grade fever and elevated sedimentation rate. Definitive diagnosis is made with a temporal artery biopsy, which is not something you rush out and do to everyone with a bad headache. Because it is inflammatory, Prednisone is the drug of choice, which is not something you rush out and do to everyone with a bad headache, either.

It is the temporal artery that feeds the rods and cones in the retina of the eye. Some people get their diagnosis made by the ophthalmologist they are sent to because their vision is changing – anywhere on the continuum of mild change to blind in that eye.

Primary and Secondary Headaches

Primary Headaches
- Migraine
- Cluster
- Muscle contraction
- Miscellaneous, not associated with a structural lesion

Secondary Headaches
- Head trauma
- Vascular disorders
- Nonvascular inter-cranial disorder
- Substance use or withdrawal
- Non-cephalic infection
- Metabolic disorder
- Disorder of cranium, facial or cranial structure
- Neuralgia, nerve trunk pain

Headaches can have a primary cause such as migraine, muscle contraction, or structural lesions. In these events, the headache is a direct reflection of the event. Some headaches, however, are secondary to other things. For example, getting hit on your head can cause a headache. Vascular disorders and substance use or withdrawal (most notably caffeine) can cause headaches. Infections in places other than your head (that empyema in your chest or the non-healing ulcer on your foot) via toxins, or metabolic disorders like having your electrolytes, BUN and Cr, or liver enzymes out of balance can cause headaches. Anything that keeps your spinal fluid from draining as it should, disorders of the cranium, facial or cranial structure, and neuralgia and nerve trunk pain can also cause headaches.

Key Components in Chapter 6

1. Our patients are sicker than they have ever been before, so the chances a headache is a serious problem is greater than it has ever been before.

2. Asking whether or not a headache is the same as usual or if it is different is crucial information no matter what the patient just complained about. Remember to grab quick neuro signs to prove whether or not there has been a change.

3. If anything is different from the patient's usual and accustomed headache, it requires a physician. Remember to always, always ask the questions.

Chapter 7

The Look Test

If someone says to you that your patient doesn't look right, what do they mean? Maybe you just "feel" something isn't quite as it should be. What is this thing called nurse's intuition? Nurses knew they had intuition, but they didn't know how to describe it until two nurses, Benner and Tanner, did a study. They discovered that a nurse's "intuition" was rapid critical thinking based on his or her past experience. In other words, every time you had ever seen a patient look that way or act that way, nothing good had ever come of it! That is your intuition, and this is also why novices *have* no such thing because they have no past experience.

When we talk about how a patient *looks*, what things are we discussing? The following has been compiled with the help of many nurses, with many, many, many years of experience. These nurses were asked to tell me the clues they had noticed over the years that indicated a patient isn't doing very well. The result is

The Look Test.

- Color
- Effort – Fatigability
- Skin – Diaphoresis
- Change in mentation
- ↑ HR ↓ RR
- Frightened ("Don't leave me")

One of the first things you notice about patients is their color. Skin color is a factor of pigmentation into the skin and oxygenation and perfusion within the capillary bed. People are not supposed to change color. They are to stay the color God gave them, and if they start changing color it's a very bad sign because that means they are not oxygenating and perfusing as well as they should. I once watched a patient in the ER turn a rainbow of colors, never realizing that that change in color was heralding his imminent cardiac arrest. If your patient changes color, it is a sign of bad things – like a failure to oxygenate and perfuse at the same time, leading to a lethal dysrythmia. You are not supposed to change colors!

We didn't used to care much if a patient was breathing really fast to keep his O2 Sat at 97%. We were just happy he had a sat of 97%. Well, we now care a great deal about the effort the patient is putting out to keep his numbers where they are because we recognize fatigability to be a real crisis generator. How hard is the patient working to keep those numbers up? How long do you think he will be able to keep going?

I know a doctor who says the worst thing we ever did was to invent the O2 sat monitor, because people stopped looking at the patient. How hard the patient is working to keep those numbers where they are is crucial information.

We now recognize diaphoresis to be a sign of maximal sympathetic stimulation and as such, a sign of impending doom. Diaphoresis is a sympathetic response that uses a parasympathetic neurotransmitter. Why do you care? Because anyone who is diaphoretic is maximally sympathetically stimulated. One more little *anything* and the patient crashes and burns. A diaphoretic patient is a ticking time bomb.

Subtle changes in mentation may mean that this patient is not oxygenating and perfusing quite as well as he was before. One day at work, a patient told me a story about something that had happened in the news that day. Four hours later, he told me the same story again. His temperature was up a bit, not much, but it was the subtle change in mentation that made me look at him again. The septic workup proved his early sepsis.

Or maybe the heart rate and respiratory rate are increasing, but there isn't any other change. The heart rate and respiratory rate climbing are your first two compensatory mechanisms the body will use to make things better. When these mechanisms fail, then we get the symptoms we learned in school about the signs of illness, which are the heart rate and respiratory rate going up. But again, you must be looking at trends, or you will never see it.

We have all experienced the patient who appears frightened and says, *"Don't leave me!"* or the ever-popular, *"I think I'm going to die!"* You are very aware of how things are going in your body at all times. You know your lytes, blood sugar, O2 sat, etc., etc. And these things are fine. You take the information and put it into your subconscious because you have a life to live, and you can't deal with the information on a minute by minute basis.

This information on your body's functioning stays in the recesses of your conscious until something goes wrong. Then it comes immediately to the forefront and gives you a sympathetic stimulation, which is what causes this patient's frightened, wide-eyed, and agitated appearance. Anyone who says to you, *"Don't leave me!"* is trying to tell you they have had that sympathetic stimulation. They probably can't tell you what is wrong, just that something is definitely not right. They are trying to warn you that they are receiving a sub-clinical sign of their impending doom.

Pay attention to people who tell you they aren't going to make it through this event. I know a surgeon who won't operate if a patient tells him they don't feel like they are going to make it. He's had too many people die after telling him that. You are much more attuned to your body than you think you are. Some people seem to know when they are going to die. Nurses see it over and over again. Pay attention.

- Eyes
- Smell
- Nurse just senses something's not right

People's eyes sparkle. The sparkle-o-meter runs from +4 sparkle to dull and glazed over. On any given day, you and I sparkle at about a +3. You make it to +4 if you are happy or delighted and, if you are getting sick, your eyes don't sparkle quite as much as they used to. You may have noticed in your children that before they give you concrete signs that indeed they are headed into another ear infection, strep throat, or whatever, their eyes don't sparkle as much they usually do.

Did you know that there are people who can smell a patient getting ready to code? *What?! Smell a patient getting ready to code?* You know we have animals that can be trained to detect lots of things. We have bomb-sniffing, cadaver, and rescue dogs. There are animals that have been trained to sense when their master is getting ready to have a seizure. The animal gives a signal and the owner lies down so they don't fall down and hurt themselves. Animals that can sense when a diabetic's blood sugar is dropping off precipitously, give a signal and the owner checks their blood sugar.

"But," you say, *"Those are animals."* Well, guess what, we are animals too, and who says we can't smell or sense a lot of what other animals do. Just like dogs and other animals, some humans smell and sense better than other humans. I, personally, can't smell acetone breath. Other people are gagging in the hallway and I'm like, *"What?"* Turns out smelling acetone breath is genetic. Forty-five percent of us cannot smell it.

All the diseases have their own distinctive aromas. All the infections also have their own distinctive aromas. No one taught us what we were smelling when we were in school because we have lab tests, but healthcare workers in Third World countries are taught to smell the differences in diseases, and the difference in infections. It was never deemed important for us to learn what smells indicate, but over time you have probably learned associations. Can you smell cancer on a patient? C-diff? Pseudomonas? Strep throat? See, you smell it too.

When I ask people who say they can smell a patient getting ready to code what it smells like, overwhelmingly I get the same answer. The first response is, *"Well.....ummm... it's hard to describe."* Apparently it is a very distinctive, very unpleasant smell like no other. If you push further, the nurse will describe it as a very unpleasant sweet, musty smell. Like socks that have been in the gym bag at school for a year. One nurse said it reminds her of rancid body odor, but that it is a distinctive odor unto itself. Another said it smelled earthy, like mushrooms.

Just like animals vary in their ability to smell, so do humans. Some nurses claim to smell patients with electrolyte imbalances or fluid overload. Every disease has its own particular smell; we just weren't ever taught what we smelled. Do animals sense more than we do? I think we just don't pay attention to what we sense. We get "feelings' about situations, but we ignore the information because we are looking for things we can talk to the doctor about – concrete signs, not "feelings." Those feelings are a large part of nurse's intuition. Pay attention to them. If you feel uneasy, respect that in yourself. It is valuable data.

- Family
- Voice
- Change in activity level
- Preoccupied
- Picking

Nursing school is full of family – the support of family, the joy and wonder of family, and all we want is for them to go home. *"He's feeling better now. Why don't you go home? There's nothing more you can do for him. Why don't you go home?"* All said with the best of intentions, but when the family leaves, so does the history of that patient and that patient's support group. Do you think unconscious people are aware of people around them? Maybe, yes? Try your best to include the family. I know it increases the stress involved in taking care of the patient, but it is the family who knows what this person is supposed to walk like, talk like, and provides the emotional support for the patient. There are exceptions, of course, where the family is a negative factor, but not that often.

The trouble with family is that we tend to think of them as ignorant and in the way. Have you ever noticed that when you are standing at the bedside as the nurse, you're pretty smart? But, as soon as you sit down at your mother's bedside, you become brain dead? The health care staff are the keepers of the knowledge, and the families are the lucky recipients of our collective wisdom if they obey the rules and are lucky.

Over the years we have gotten much, much better at including family at the bedside. We still have a way to go in learning to listen to them when they tell us Uncle George isn't looking or behaving in his normal way. Listen to the family! They know these people; we don't. Teach your novice to listen to the patient.

If the patient says it's not right, it's not right. If the family says it's not right, it's not right. All morning long a patient's wife tried to tell a non-responsive nurse that this was not normal behavior for her husband. The nurse paid no attention. After the patient coded, the wife was in the hallway screaming, *"Do you believe me now?!"* Listen to the patient and his family!

You can tell a great deal about people from their voices. You can tell oxygenation and perfusion from the strength of the voice and clarity of ideas. You can also tell tidal volume from someone's voice. It has to do with the number of words you can string together in a sentence. If you can string a bunch of them together, you have good volume. If you start making very short, succinct sentences or taking a breath every few words, your tidal volume and / or oxygenation is decreasing. I had a telephone triage nurse tell me she could hear sympathetic stimulation in a patient's voice. She said it sounds like fear. I bet it does.

Any patient who has had a sudden change in activity level is talking to you. That can be the antsy patient who is suddenly calm or the calm patient who is suddenly antsy. There has been a change and you need to come see about the patient.

The patient who was preoccupied as you were walking around his room is not normal. He should be paying close attention to you. If he's not, he's not oxygenating and perfusing quite as well as he was before. Look for what has changed.

The first sign of a change in behavior that I learned when I was in school is "picking". What are they picking at? Everything; the air, their bedclothes, their dressing; they just want to re-tape their IV onto the bedrail so you can get at it easier. Would they please just leave things alone? Have you, yourself, ever been confused? You know things aren't real, but maybe they are. What is real and what isn't? You don't want to be confused and you sure don't want to let anyone know you don't know exactly what is going on. Try to be a kind as you can to your confused patient (every nurse's favorite patient). It isn't their fault and they will be better as soon as they can.

- The numbers don't add up
- Having "a better day"
- Visits from the dead
- Sees a religious figure
- Hungry at an odd time

Vital signs fit together in groups. Good, bad, or ugly, they fit into their assigned group. But, what if you get a number that doesn't seem to fit? You have a patient who is blue, with respiratory rate and heart rate both up, but the O2 sat is 98%. What do you do? Retake your numbers, look for variables and if things are still not adding up, ask for what I like to call a *nursing consult*. A nursing consult is where you turn to the nurse next to you and say, "*What do you think?*" Some of us seem to think that we can't ask for help because it will show our lack of knowledge and decrease our status. But if you look at your best nurses, they are always turning to each other and saying, "*What do you think?*" The highest form of nursing is one practiced with lots of nursing consults. The lowest form of nursing is the "lone ranger" approach.

Turn to the nurse next to you; turn to the clinician next to you. Whether it is dietary, respiratory, physical therapy, social services – these people have a wealth of knowledge we do not possess. The more people you involve in your decision, the better your chances of having a good outcome. Use the team approach.

When you look at numbers, always ask yourself, "*Who generated this number?*" Nurse's aides frequently generate numbers that the nurse acts upon. If a number is not fitting into its grouping – go take it yourself. If you send the nurse's aide back to retake it, she might simply make the same mistake again.

Some nurse's aides have received very poor education in how to take a pulse oximetry reading. You'll see them go into the patient's room, slip the probe onto the finger, and turn the machine on. They take the very first number that pops up – particularly if it is a good number! – whip the probe off the finger and they are out the door before the machine ever gets a chance to equate itself. As you well know, if the patient's *current* apical heart rate (not what it was a 0830 this morning) is not correlated to the heart rate on the machine, or you have a very brisk pleth, the number is garbage.

It is also considered cheating to hyperventilate the patient into a good number! *"Bertha take a breath! That's good. Do it again. OK, deeper, deeper. One more time. That's good!"* And you whip the probe off the finger, and out the door you go while Bertha once again hypoventilates. You want the number to reflect where the patient is, not where you occasionally stimulate them to be.

Watch the patient who is suddenly having a better day. You could be looking at the last catecholamine surge where the body takes everything it has left and summons up one last effort to stay alive. This is the patient who has been sick as a dog, who one morning sits up, eats with a good appetite, has a lovely chat with relatives, and dies the next day. Nurses see this over and over again.

Visits from the dead can be a very bad sign. If you work in an extended care facility, you are happy to see dead people show up because they entertain your patients. They talk about the old days, take your patient out to eat, gossip about the family. But the one place you don't want to see dead people show up is at an acute care crisis. The patient's husband has been dead for six years. Now he is sitting on the end of the bed talking to her. This is a very bad sign. He has probably come to take her with him down the tunnel.

Seeing a religious figure is also bad. (The patient, not the nurse seeing a religious figure. You should not be having religious visions at work. If you are, please go home and come back later.) I use the phrase "see a religious figure" because it depends on the patient's religion as to what figure they might see. If the patient is Christian and looks up and starts talking to Jesus or to angels, the situation is deteriorating rapidly.

Pay attention to the patient who is hungry at an odd time. A Type II diabetic on oral diabetic medications has been admitted to the hospital to have cardiac meds started up. It is 1 o'clock in the afternoon. He calls his nurse and says, "*I'm hungry. Can I have something to eat?*" The nurse says, "*Why are you hungry? You just had lunch and you ate everything on your tray. I know because I picked it up.*" To which the patient replied, "*I don't know. I'm just hungry. OK? Can I get something to eat?*"

What this nurse knew was that when a diabetic's blood glucose is dropping, there is a zone at which, no matter when the person last put food in their mouth, he becomes hungry. Knowing this, she checked the patient's blood glucose and it was 45. The patient was having a reaction between his oral diabetic medication and his new cardiac medication, but it was being hungry at an odd time that tripped the nurse to it. The blood glucose was ordered half an hour before meals and at bedtime. How would this patient have been if the nurse had waited until 1630 to check the blood sugar? Dead. Do not hesitate to get a blood glucose on a diabetic patient.

This zone of hunger has a bottom to it. If a diabetic ever asks for something to eat and you can't get it to them right away, and you go back later and the diabetic claims to no longer be hungry – check the blood glucose. That zone of hunger has a bottom to it, and if the patient doesn't eat he can fall right out of the hunger zone into the "I'm in big trouble zone" while still

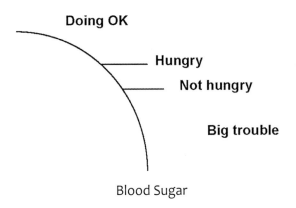

129

appearing to be just fine because all they are doing is lying in bed. We tend to think that if the patient is talking to us, the sugar can't be too bad. What is the lowest blood sugar you have had on a patient who is talking to you? Forty? Thirty? Twenty?!

- Ear and nose cartilage relaxes
- Heavenward gaze in unconscious pt.
- Blue knees
- The patient who is afraid of going to bed

Some nurses have noticed that before a patient dies, the ear and nose cartilage relaxes. Your ears are firm and stick out from the sides of your head. Because of this, they are ideal for supporting nasal cannula. Right before death, because of oxygenation and perfusion – and the lack thereof – the cartilage becomes soft. Some nurses say the ears lay back against the head. Others say they curl up from the bottom or curl down from the tops, but you noticed it happening when you can't keep the nasal cannula on the patient's ears and you had to start taping it to the patient's cheeks. The nose also gets very doughy and if you are trying to put an O2 mask on the patient, it keeps slipping and you end up taping it to his cheeks.

When you have an unconscious patient, every few hours you do neuro checks where you look at the patient's pupils. You open the eyes to shine your light into the pupils and the eyes are right there looking back at you. The next time you come along and raise the eyelids you see that the eyes have rolled back in the patient's head. That is the heavenward gaze in the unconscious patient, indicating that things have deteriorated.

Mottling anywhere in your body is a bad idea, and one of the first places patients mottle is the kneecaps. Blue knees are a bad sign.

Then there are the patients who won't go to bed. It is like they know that if they get in the bed, lie down, and go to sleep, they are going to die. Now, that's silly, isn't it? People don't know when they are going to die, do they? Many nurses will say, *"Yes, they do."*

Some patients seem to have a premonition of their deaths and contact family members for a last chat before they pass on unexpectedly.

- Can't get O2 Saturation any more
- Can't hold body temperature
- Soles of feet in a code
- Craving ice
- Last face

The pulse oximetry that had been working just fine no longer seems able to find the patient's pulse, and it keeps alarming. Some nurses have been known to turn off the alarms thinking it was a machine malfunction. But what's happening is that perfusion is decreasing into that extremity. *Check the patient!*

When a patient can't hold his body temperature up, that is another sign of impending doom. This spells poor oxygenation and perfusion in your patient, because the body's thermostat is located in the brain.

A nurse told me that she could tell if a patient was going to make it through a code based on the color of the soles of his feet. If the feet were gray or alabaster white, he wasn't going to make it, and if they were somewhere between the two extremes, he *might* make it. Again, I bet it has to do with the degree of oxygenation and circulatory shutdown.

What is the patient who craves ice trying to tell you? She could be anemic. Anemics are well known to crave ice. This is called ice pica. (Why they crave ice, I have no idea, they just do. If any of you know the pathophysiology behind this phenomena, I sure would like to know.) It isn't the contents of the ice – you could get that by drinking water. It has something to do with the crunch.

Another group that craves ice are people whose tanks are empty. If all the nurse will give them is ice chips, they will take gallons of ice and try to fill their tanks back up. This is why some post-op, hemorrhaging, or trauma patients crave ice.

The term "last face" comes from a paramedic who says she just hates it when the patient says, "*You are the last face I am going to see,"* because invariably this statement came true. She has had it happen to her several times. It is, again, a premonition of death that some patients clearly have.

- Black dog

We have done very little study of end of life experiences. If the patient sees something we don't see, we assume they are confused and hallucinating. But, what if a lot of patients see the *same* hallucination? I have been told of numerous incidences where nurses were told by patients that they saw a black dog in their rooms before they died. One nurse learned of the black dog when her patient said, *"I didn't know you allowed pets in the ICU."* The nurse said, *"What pet?"* And the patient replied, *"That black dog over in the corner."*

The very interesting thing about the black dog is that the patients frequently reported seeing the same black dog. It is the size of a German shepherd or a lab with medium length black hair. It has been reported to be in the corner, under the bed, on the bed, or outside a window looking in at the patient. Its presence is usually benign, and the patients don't mind it being there. One patient slept with her arm around the dog. Another one reported that the dog came running up to him, put his head on his lap, and looked up at him adoringly. All these patients died.

Not every dying patient sees the black dog, but some do. What is the significance of the black dog? It appears in religious myths from all around the world, and it always has to do with the death experience. We have done very little study into end of life experiences, and here is some nursing research just waiting to happen.

Key Components in Chapter 7

1. Intuition is your past experience talking to you. Honor it and act.
2. How the patient looks and how hard he is working are vastly more important than numbers on a machine.
3. Listen to what your patient is saying, the words he uses, the number of words in a sentence and if he sounds frightened.
4. Look under the covers at the whole patient.
5. Use the clinicians around you to help you make good decisions.

Chapter 8

Renal

Functions of the Kidneys
- Eliminate metabolic waste
    - urea
    - creatinine
    - uric acid
- Regulate extracellular volume
- Osmolality of body fluids
- Electrolyte balance
- Acid-base balance
- Secrete hormones
    - renin
    - erythropoietin
    - prostaglandins
- gluconeogenesis
    - glucose from amino acids

Your kidneys are responsible for excreting the waste products of your metabolic functioning. They regulate volume and osmolality of the body's fluids. They balance electrolytes and pH, secrete hormones, and are capable of gluconeogenesis.

Now, I want you to believe that the kidneys regulate your blood pressure and your hematocrit That would make no sense at all if you had discrete organ systems that functioned independently of the other organs. But you don't. You have one set of completely interrelated organs. So of course the kidneys can regulate your blood pressure, gastric mucosa and hematocrit if they want to.

The kidneys are also capable of gluconeogenesis – making new sugar from amino acids. In a time of crisis, like shock, they can scrape together the components of ATP and try to keep themselves alive. This shows you how important they are to the body.

Renal Function Studies

BUN	Creatinine	Diagnosis
⬆	Normal or slightly ↑	Volume depletion or Poor perfusion
⬆	Normal or slightly ↑	Protein catabolism
⬆	⬆	Kidney disease

When you look at someone's kidney function, you look at the BUN and Creatinine (Cr). If both the BUN and Cr are both up, you have someone with renal dysfunction. But there are two other things that make the BUN go up, but not the Cr. The first one, you see all the time: volume depletion. A little old lady comes in dehydrated, and her BUN is high. You rehydrate her, and in the next day or so her BUN falls to normal. This is a concentration issue. Low perfusion through the kidney from whatever reason also allows BUN to build up in the circulatory system

The other group that has a high BUN without renal failure are patients who have a lot of protein to metabolize. Earlier, we said an end product of protein metabolism was BUN. Patients with crushing injuries have a lot of myoglobin to metabolize to protein and excrete, as do burn and trauma patients. Patients with red blood cells out of the blood vessels but still within their body – hematomas, GI bleeds, trauma, etc. – have large amounts of protein to be metabolized. With these patients you expect to see the BUN go up as the protein is broken down for the excretion process – but not the Cr. When both are up you have kidney problems.

Is He Wet or Is He Dry?

Fluid depletion
- tachycardia
- variable BP
- ↓ urine output
- dry mucus membranes
- ↑ thirst

Fluid overload
- tachycardia
- variable BP
- ↓ urine output
- rales
- edema
- hypoxia, dyspnea
- JVD

Is he wet or is he dry? How do you tell? The answer to this question drove Drs. William Ganz and Jeremy Swan to invent their famous catheter in the 1970s. When the first Swan-Ganz catheters came out, they came with a questionnaire asking the doctor to guess whether they thought the patient was wet or dry. Then, they were to put the catheter in and tell the researchers what numbers they got. What they found was that 50% of the time the doctor guessed wrong. But why can't you tell?

The problem is the signs and symptoms. The first three are identical for both groups. Heart rate goes up because stroke volume falls off both when you are over-loaded and under-loaded, so that is not an indicator. Because of vasoconstriction, blood pressure is not a good indicator. Both groups also stop making urine. So how do you know?

You can rely on thirst as an indicator of volume depletion *only* if you have a patient with an intact thirst mechanism and the ability to ask for a glass of water. You don't always get that. If you live long enough, everything in your body is going to fail you including your thirst mechanism. No one has to tell young people to go get a drink. They have brisk thirst mechanisms, but as you get older the thirst mechanism loses its briskness. This is why little, old people so often end up in the hospital with dehydration. They don't know to take a drink. If you work with these people, you must constantly offer them something to drink whether they want it or not.

But you can tell if a patient is overhydrated, can't you, because they have crackles, edema, shortness of breath, and hypoxia, right? But crackles, edema, shortness of breath, and hypoxia can each be caused by many other things, and they are not characteristic only to fluid overload.

The only useful sign of overhydration is jugular venous distention (JVD). In the absence of right heart failure, it is JVD that tells you this patient is fluid overloaded. You can call the doctor and describe low oxygen saturations, rapid heart rates, swollen ankles, and wet lungs – but all of those signs can have multiple causes. The things that can cause positive JVD are constrictive pericarditis, inferior vena cava obstruction, severe tricuspid regurgitation, cardiac tamponade, massive pulmonary embolus, superior vena

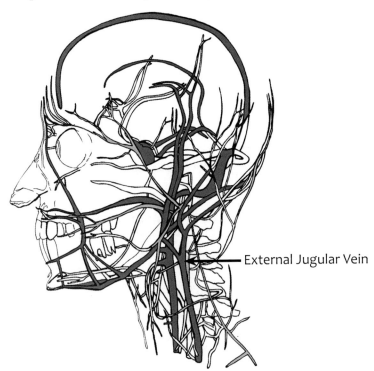

External Jugular Vein

Figure 8-1. External Jugular Vein

cava syndrome, right heart failure, and fluid overload. The ones you are most likely to run into are right heart failure and fluid overload. In the absence of right heart failure, the most likely cause of positive JVD is fluid overload.

Most nurses don't know how to measure JVD, so let me explain.

What you are looking for is the external jugular vein that runs up the side of the neck. You have the patient at a 30 – 45 degree elevation (depending on which author you read) at rest in bed, feet up. Then you look to see if you can see the vein. It's not a "can I palpate," it is a "can I see" thing. If you have a patent with a fat neck you may need to turn the head or pull the skin. If you have an extremely thin patient, they are little anatomy lessons just laying there and you may always see their veins. But, for the average patient this will work just fine.

All right, we have the patient in bed, the head of the bed up 45 degrees, and we look to see if the vein can be seen. If you can see it, how many finger widths does it take to cover it up? JVD is measured in + 1, +2, +3, or +4 and the pluses represent the width of your fingers when they are held parallel to the ground. Plus one means it took the width of one finger placed horizontally to cover the vein, plus three means it took three finger widths, etc. The zero point is the top of the patient's clavicle. Find the top of the clavicle, look for the vein, see how many fingers it takes to cover it over, put a + sign in front of how many fingers it took, and there is your measurement.

Zero to +1 is normal. You cannot see fluid deficit because the vein falls down into the chest and most of us can't see into the chest, so JVD is good for fluid overload only. You will see doctors check JVD on patients sitting up in chairs. If you have positive JVD sitting up, you definitely have positive JVD in bed at a 45 degree angle. Patients in fluid overload are frequently in respiratory distress and sitting up lowers the amount of blood returning into the heart (preload) thereby decreasing CHF symptoms. Asking the patient to get into bed, put their feet on the bed, and their head down to a 45 degree angle can precipitate a respiratory and / or cardiac crisis. If they don't have positive JVD sitting up, it doesn't mean they won't have it at a 45 degree angle in bed. One does not preclude the other in this case.

Key Components in Chapter 8

1. You have one set of completely interrelated organs – not distinct, separate systems.
2. A high BUN can mean poor perfusion into the kidney or a lot of protein that needs to be metabolized and excreted.
3. When both the BUN and Cr are up, the patient has renal issues.
4. In the absence of right heart failure, it is a positive JVD that tells you that your patient is fluid overloaded.

Chapter 9

The Effects of Surgical Trauma

The Body's Regulatory Systems

- Autoregulation GFR
- RAAS
- Aldosterone
- Antidiuretic hormone
- Baroreceptors
- Volume receptors
- Atrial natriuretic factor
- Osmoreceptors

Autoregulation

The name of the game is homeostasis, and the body has all kinds of regulatory systems designed to keep you in homeostasis. The first one on the list is something called autoregulation within the capillary beds. Your capillaries are one cell thick at their smallest. This is a very fragile system. If every time your blood pressure went up because you were scared, angry, excited, whatever – if that increase in pressure had been transmitted into those capillaries, you would have blown them all apart by now. When you go to sleep, your blood pressure drops and flow in the capillaries slows. When blood slows down, it tends to clot. It is *supposed* to, but it can make getting out of bed in the morning very difficult!

We need a method for mediating blood flow through the capillaries, and we have one called autoregulation. *Dorland's Medical Dictionary* defines autoregulation as:

1. The process occurring when some mechanism within a biological system detects and adjusts for changes within the system; exercised by negative feedback.
2. In circulatory physiology, the intrinsic tendency of an organ or tissue to maintain constant blood flow despite changes in arterial pressure, or the adjustment of blood flow through an organ in order to provide for its metabolic needs.

Pre- and Post-Capillary Sphincters

We have pre- and post-capillary bed sphincters that respond to various chemicals and metabolic events. They open and close the sphincters and regulate blood flow through the capillaries based on the needs of the cells they service.

Capillary Bed

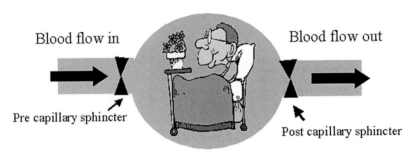

Blood flow in

Blood flow out

Pre capillary sphincter

Post capillary sphincter

By opening and closing the sphincters, it is possible to protect the delicate capillary bed from systolic pressures up to 180 mm Hg and all the way down to a systolic pressure of 80 mm Hg. The same degree of flow can be maintained throughout this continuum. Here's how it works. If the arterial pressure is increasing, you constrict the pre-capillary sphincter to reduce the pressure into the capillary bed while at the same time you open the post-capillary sphincter to let the pressure out the other side. Physiologists think this process is driven not only by stretch receptors, but also by the metabolic need of the tissues fed by this capillary.

The system also works in reverse. If the arterial pressure is dropping, the pre-capillary sphincter opens while the post-capillary one closes. This increases the pressure within the capillary bed. It can also cause capillary sludging where flow slows in the affected capillaries and the clotting cascade is activated. This is a wonderful way to get disseminated intravascular coagulopathy (DIC). It is important to keep the patient's pressure up to prevent DIC.

The autoregulation mentioned in the caption says "GFR." That refers to the glomeral filtration rate in the kidney.

Autoregulation protects the delicate nephron and its capillary from damage from systolic pressures up to 180 mm Hg and all the way down to a systolic pressure of 80 mm Hg. This way, the patient can continue to make urine over a wide range of blood pressures and be protected from the spikes in blood pressure that go with everyday living.

RAAS

Simply put, the renin angiotensin aldosterone system (RAAS) is a method for maintaining blood volume during a time of trauma. It is left over from the caveman days, right along with the autonomic nervous system. Let's say you were attacked by a saber-tooth tiger, and you are now bleeding profusely. Let's vasoconstrict the blood vessels, because vasoconstriction helps keep perfusion pressures up.and it is easier to clot off a small hole Next, you don't want to continue making urine at the same rate as before the trauma, because if you do, you won't manage to hang on to all your remaining volume. Finally, if you crawled over to the creek and drank a lot of water, would that help with your blood volume problem? Yes, it would. The end products of the RAAS are that it is a very potent vasoconstrictor, it makes you retain sodium and water, and it activates your thirst mechanism.

The renin angiotensin aldosterone system (RAAS) is a marvel. The kidneys don't know that they aren't part of the cardiovascular system. When blood flows into the kidney, it measures the pressure with something called the justaglomeral apparatus. If the pressure is down, it causes the kidney to secrete rennin, which goes out into the circulation looking for the angiotensinogen that was placed there by the liver. The two combine and turn themselves into angiotensin I, which goes rushing off to the lungs looking for the angiotensin converting enzyme, finds it, and turns itself in angiotensin II.

Angiotensin II has multiple effects in the body, but there are two effects in particular that we are interested in:

1. It goes off to the brain, causes the release of ACTH, which goes to the adrenal gland causing the secretion of aldosterone, which goes to the kidney causing the renal tubule to retain sodium and water, and

2. it is a very potent vasoconstrictor.

We just whipped our way through seven organ systems regulating your blood pressure. You do not have multiple sets of independent organ systems, you have *one set* of interrelated organs.

Antidiuretic Hormone

Another regulatory mechanism is the antidiuretic hormone (ADH). It is activated when there appears to be a need to retain water within the body, as with cases of stress, increased sodium levels, or hypotension. The stress response itself can cause the secretion of aldosterone and the retention of sodium and water by the kidneys. This is designed to increase blood volume at a time of stress, which would increase transport capacity and reserve.

Baroreceptors

There are little pressure plates called baroreceptors throughout the body measuring the blood pressure. There is a concentration of them in the arch of the aorta. They talk to the autonomic nervous system via sympathetic and parasympathetic nerve fibers. Homeostasis wants a nice even blood pressure – no spikes, no troughs. As the blood leaves the left ventricle and goes out into the aorta, the baroreceptors measure the blood pressure. If the pressure is going up, the body decreases the heart rate and vasodilates a little bit. If the pressure is going down, it increases the heart rate and vasoconstricts the blood vessels a bit. In this way, you keep a nice even blood pressure. If the vascular volume is also dropping, it causes the secretion of ADH which in turn causes the kidneys to retain water and increases blood pressure. Stimulating the parasympathetic side of the autonomic nervous system causes what is known as a vaso-vagal response, which causes a precipitous drop in the heart rate and blood pressure.

Conversely, stimulating the sympathetic side of the autonomic nervous system causes the heart rate and blood pressure to increase. Homeostasis wants a balance.

Volume and Stretch Receptors

There are volume and stretch receptors in the atria of the heart. The atria also contain stretch receptors. When the atria are stretched by volume overload, these receptors cause the atria to secrete atrial natriuretic factor. The released peptide acts on the renal tubule, causing an excretion of sodium and water. When the volume load goes down, the receptors return to normal. And, of course, there are the ever-popular osmoreceptors that are tied directly into the thirst mechanism.

The Effects of Surgical Trauma

The previous regulatory systems are simply the ones that we know about today. Tomorrow, I'm sure we will know of more. What we want to look at next is what happens to these regulatory systems if you sign the op permit; the effects of surgical trauma. Surgery is indeed trauma. It is *scheduled* trauma, but the effect is the same.

Surgery's Effect on the Regulatory Mechanisms

General anesthesia
- narcotics – vasodilators
- succinylcholine – increase K+ levels
- sedatives and muscle relaxants – decrease myocardial contractility
- blunt compensatory mechanisms a minimum of 24 hours (the longer the surgery, the longer the effect)
- Blood and fluid loss → RAAS
- Third space fluid shifts
- Mechanical ventilation
- Hypothermia

If a patient gets a general anesthesia with your surgery and receives narcotics like Fentanyl, these vasodilators can cause pressure and volume problems. The succinylcholine given to paralyze the patient so the ET tube can be inserted increases potassium levels by pulling potassium out of the cell into the serum. Anesthetic gasses, sedatives, and muscle relaxants decrease myocardial contractility. If a healthy person's myocardial contractility is decreased, it isn't a big problem because healthy young people have lots of reserves. But do you operate on sweet young things or old geezers and geezerettes? Decreasing some of your patient's myocardial contractility can cause you to wish you had never come to work that day, because the regulatory mechanisms are blunted for a minimum of 24 hours (the longer the surgery, the longer the effect). Also, the more co-morbid factors going into the surgery and the more complications post-op, the longer the blunt.

When patients bleed from surgery, they will set off their renin angiotensin aldosterone system to minimize the decrease in vascular volume and blood pressure. Patients achieve this by retaining sodium and water in their kidneys and by vasoconstriction of the blood vessels. If the patient retains sodium and water, it makes the preload in the heart go up – a bad idea in a patient with heart failure. Vasoconstriction makes the afterload of the heart go up – also a bad idea in a heart failure patient. Both of those normal compensatory mechanisms increase the workload of the heart. For the patient with heart failure, the surgical incision is a double whammy.

Being on a ventilator can increase volumes within the chest, activating baro and volume receptors, stimulating the RAAS and ADH secretion, leading to an increase of sodium and water. You can get Syndrome of Inappropriate Antidiuretic Hormone (SIADH) simply by being placed on a ventilator.

The hypothermia the patient comes out of the OR with decreases in his metabolic needs, but this also decreases myocardial contractility, drops the heart rate, causes peripheral vasoconstriction (raising the workload of the heart), impairs insulin release, and stimulates the RAAS. This can cause hypertension, hyperglycemia, decreased cardiac output, and fluid and electrolyte imbalance. Not your favorite things to have happen to your elderly and/or frail patient.

The Effects of Surgical Trauma
12 to 48 hrs post insult
- vascular depletion
- dry mucus membranes
- edema
- weight gain
- ↑ serum glucose
- ↓ K+
- cool pale skin
- irregular HR

When the surgeon takes the knife and makes an incision into the skin, it is an injury. It is no different than if you accidentally cut yourself. You set off the response to injury, the capillaries vasodilate, the slit pores open up, and out goes the fluid. Because of this, you are now volume depleted. This is why they give your patient so much fluid in surgery and recovery. They are trying to fill the patient's tank back up. Unfortunately, you can overfill the tank, throwing the patient into CHF. It is sometimes a delicate balance.

Because the slit pores opened up and the fluid poured out, your patient is edematous. Edema is no indicator of fluid overload in the post-op patient – they are *all* edematous because of the response to injury. This is also why patients gain weight post-op. Each liter of fluid weighs 2.2 pounds (or 1 Kg depending on the system you are using).

Because of the stress response and your glucocorticoids, your serum glucose is abnormal. Because of the stress response and the minerocorticoids, the electrolytes are abnormal. These are two of the four things (normal pH, balanced electrolytes, oxygen and glucose inside the cell being used to make ATP) that can lead to a lethal dysrythmia. This is a delicate situation requiring an observant nurse.

24 to 72 hours post insult (reabsorption/diuresis phase)
- decreased capillary permeability
- decreased third spacing
- increased vascular volume
- Na+ excess
- K+ depletion

Your patient has survived the immediate post-op period, and she is going home tomorrow. You are looking at making out assignments for the night shift. Can you give her to the weakest nurse on the floor? Yes, you do. You have to give him someone; you can't take care of the whole floor. Besides, she is going home tomorrow. What could go wrong?

Our patient hasn't felt too well today, but she just had major surgery – how well are you supposed to feel? She does know if she sits in a chair, on the side of the bed, or walks around pushing her IV pole, she actually feels better. So she has done this all day, which has convinced you that this patient is ready to go home.

At 2100, the nurse comes in and gives her a sleeping pill. Now within minutes to hours, depending on the strength of her compensatory mechanism, all the blood she was pooling in her legs while she was upright is going to be thrown back into the circulatory system. Then her preload will go up and she'll go right into congestive heart failure.

Where did all the fluid come from? Remember those capillaries that dilated in response to injury/inflammation? Remember the slit pores that opened up and all the fluid that poured out? Well, at some point post-op, those slit pores are going to close up again, and when they do, all that fluid out in the periphery will get picked up and pulled back into the vascular space, increasing the preload in the heart. If you are young and healthy, you get rid of it when you urinate. But if you are an old geezer or geezerette with a bad heart and bad lungs, you hold on to it, become fluid overloaded, go into congestive heart failure, progress to pulmonary edema, become hypoxic, have a lethal dysrythmia, and die when no one is looking at you because you are supposed to be going home tomorrow. Not exactly the outcome you were looking for.

What are the first signs that a patient is going into congestive heart failure? (Before the shortness of breath, before the numbers go bad.) Heart rate and respiratory rate begin to climb, while the urine output is less than it had been before. The only way you see it is by looking at trends. The urine output is less than it had been before, but possibly not abnormally low . . . yet. By the time the patient has overt symptoms, the compensatory mechanisms have failed.

A lot of our post-op patients are sent home before this reabsorption-diuresis phase occurs. They come back into clinics and ERs, or are discharged into extended care facilities too soon, then go into failure. The very fact that the patient is still in the hospital should be a very big clue that the doctor expects this to happen to this patient. Watch them like a hawk.

Key Components in Chapter 9

1. Surgery is scheduled trauma and it sets off inflammation system wide, just like unscheduled trauma does.

2. Increased capillary permeability causes vascular volumes to decrease which is why patients get so much fluid in surgery.

3. At some point, the capillary will close and all the fluid in the intersticium will be drawn back into the vascular space, where the patient will either pee it off or go into congestive heart failure with it.

4. The first signs of CHF are heart rate and respiratory rate starting to climb and urine output less than before. These are signs of compensation in the body. When compensation fails, we get shortness of breath, the numbers fall off, and junk in the lungs – the stuff they taught us in school.

Chapter 10

Compartment Syndrome

Compartment syndrome happens more often than not to orthopedic patients, but it also happens in a lot of other circumstances. When it hits, the results can be devastating, but are preventable if you know what you are looking for. For those reasons I have chosen to include it in this book.

All the muscle bundles in your body are wrapped in fascia. They make distinct, non-communicating compartments. The fascia is somewhat flexible – if you poke on your muscles, they gives somewhat, but they do not expand indefinitely. Because of this, they have the characteristics of a fixed space. In the illustration, we can see the four compartments of the leg. Inside the compartments are muscle, nerve, and blood vessels.

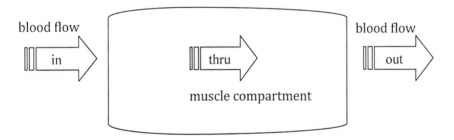

Compartment syndrome, like everything else, occurs on a continuum. You can have so little of it, we don't really need to do anything about it. Or, at the other extreme, you have it so bad you set off inflammation, SIRS, and die a horrible death on a ventilator with multiple organ failure. Let's consider the middle ground.

To have good circulation in the muscle compartment and meet the metabolic needs of the myocardial cells, the blood needs to flow into the compartment, through the compartment and out the other side. In order for this to occur, the pressure inside the compartment must never exceed the perfusion pressure.

Should the pressure inside the compartment exceed the perfusion pressure, flow into the compartment will slow and stop. This is called compartment syndrome.

There are two main pathways to allowing the pressure inside the compartment to exceed the perfusion pressure. The first one is to allow the pressure inside the compartment itself to go up – for example, if the patient bleeds into it. Other things that will do it are intensive muscle use that destroys the muscle cells resulting in rhabdomyolysis, burns, intra-arterial injections, decreased serum osmolality (i.e. nephritic syndrome), IVs infused into the compartment, venomization from snake bite, or something called "lying on limb."

In a "lying on limb" situation, the patient is so debilitated from age, illness, alcohol, or drugs that they cannot arrange their limbs in such a way that there is good blood flow in the extremities. This is the drunk who passes out with his arms over the back of a chair, or the elderly person who falls and stays in that position until help arrives to straighten her up and reestablish blood flow.

If you go to sleep at night and roll over on your arm, what happens? It hurts and wakes you up, so you turn over in order to reestablish blood flow. But what if you couldn't either wake up or turn over? The hypoxia in the muscle compartment will set off the response to injury – inflammation. The capillaries will open up, then fluid will rush out, which will raise the pressure in the compartment higher than the perfusion pressure. At this point, we'd have compartment syndrome.

Anytime that you interrupt blood flow and reestablish it later, your patient is at risk for compartment syndrome. That would include any of your vascular surgery patients and some of your orthopedic patients, like total knee replacement. It's anyone who has been in shock or had a cardiac arrest. Also at risk are patients whose NBP cuff pumped up and didn't go back down, but no one noticed it for several hours.

The second pathway into compartment syndrome is to shrink the size of the compartment while all other factors remain the same. Casting does this beautifully. Every ER used to have a fully equipped cast room. You break it, we cast it. This is no longer true. Today you are told to take this nice splint and go home. Note the Velcro closures? Loosen them if it gets tight. Come back after the swelling is gone and we will give you a nice fiberglass cast in the color of your choice. We now do it this way because of compartment syndrome.

Other things that can shrink the size of the compartment are hematomas, infiltrated IVs, and burns, particularly ones that go all the way around the limb.

So the two pathways into muscle compartment syndrome are to increase the pressure in the compartment or to shrink down the size of the compartment.

In compartment syndrome, for whatever reason, the pressure in the compartment exceeds the perfusion pressure. Because of this, blood flow into the compartment slows or stops, depending on the severity of the problem. Less oxygen is delivered to the tissues, they go anaerobic, and cannot generate the ATP they need. They become dysfunctional and begin excreting lactic acid as an end product of anaerobic metabolism. Things are not going well.

The body considers being anaerobic an injury and sets off inflammation – the response to injury. Out come the mediators, the capillaries dilate, their slit pores open up, and out goes the fluid, which in turn increases the pressure in the compartment, thereby decreasing flow into it. And around and around we go in a cycle doomed to get worse. The lactic acid excreted into the muscles hurts, and it is supposed to. It is your body's way of saying, *"Stop, stupid. We've gone anaerobic here!"* If you stop or slow your exercise rate, the pain goes away as oxygen–laden blood makes it into the cells, restoring aerobic metabolism.

If insufficient oxygen is delivered to the cells, they can't make ATP the way they should, so they can't run their Na+ - K+ - ATP pumps on the cell walls the way they should. The cells swell up, become dysfunctional, and if this goes on long enough, the cells lyse, leaving tissue necrosis in its wake. And once the cells are gone, they *never* come back again. It is not a matter of sending the patient to PT to build the muscle back up again. It is permanently gone. A patient can lose his muscle bundle, his limb, and his life. A patient can die from compartment syndrome via metabolic acidosis and/or septic shock, which may set off SIRS.

The most common place to see compartment syndrome is in the lower leg after high-velocity injuries, due to the amount of damage done to that section of the body. Possibly as many as 30% of all orthopedic cases get compartment syndrome. But remember, like everything else, compartment syndrome occurs on a continuum. You can have so little of it we hardly notice it, you can die from it, or experience any point in between these extremes.

If it is so devastating, how do you pick it up in the clinical setting? Over the years, we have taught many ways to assess patients for compartment syndrome. We taught nurses to look for pain, paraesthesia, pallor, pilothermia (burning pain), and pulselessness. However, these signs depend on having a patient who can feel and talk coherently. You don't always get that.

So how do you tell? Assuming that your patient can feel, you tell with pain. Unrelenting pain that cannot be medicated to a tolerable level should alert you to the possibility of compartment syndrome. You should be able to medicate to a tolerable level (not gone, but tolerable) any and all post-op and trauma pain. If you can't, suspect compartment syndrome. Pain should get better every day, and if it is still at the same level day after day, get suspicious.

Patients who scream and cry no matter how much pain medication they are given, or ones who have to have Narcan to reverse the all the narcotics you have been giving them trying to make them comfortable, may be trying to tell you that they have an ischemic event going on. The pain from lactic acid buildup in muscles is extreme and unrelenting until adequate blood flow is restored. When the pain stops either the muscle bundle is dead or sufficient oxygen is now present for aerobic metabolism. There is a six hour window within which to restore oxygen delivery to the muscle bundle before it becomes necrotic – never able to be revived.

If you suspect compartment syndrome, what are you going to do about it? First, if there is a cast on the extremity, get it cut off now! Do not hesitate! What if you cut a cast off and find out that compartment syndrome is not present? Have you done a bad thing? No. Somebody puts a new cast on; big deal. But if compartment syndrome is present and you didn't cut the cast off? Have you done something wrong? Oh, yes.

Remember: time is of the essence. Every minute results in more dead cells. You don't have time to page the doctor and wait around for a return call. Cut the cast off, then call the doctor and tell them what you did. You can't go wrong cutting a cast off. You can be *very* wrong if you wait. When you, or someone who knows how, cuts a cast off, remember to go all the way through the cast and down to the skin with your bandage scissors. Sometimes the wrap that was put on before the cast is the source of the stricture. By the same token, patients with only Ace wraps on their extremities can have the same problems as casted patients. If the patient has unrelenting pain, remove the wrap.

If we determine that compartment syndrome is present, what are we going to do about it? The problem is one of excessive pressure in the compartment. How bad is it really? You can insert a needle into the compartment attached to a manometer and follow the pressure. Remember, we are again on a continuum – "awful" to "not so bad." If it's "not so bad," we can try the benign neglect approach (wait and see). If it is "awful," we need to act.

What is done is something called a fasciotomy. You literally fillet the leg open down to the offending muscle bundle, slit the fascia to relieve the pressure in the bundle, and hopefully get enough perfusion going to stop the necrotic process. Fasciotomy, in the past, has meant cutting open the extremity and letting nursing students do wet to dry dressing changes in the wound. Today, we have the woundvac to aid the patient's healing, but you still start with a gaping wound.

In caring for these patients, we return to the standard of oxygenation and perfusion. If this patient has an O2 sat of 97% why does he need external oxygen? Because we are trying to

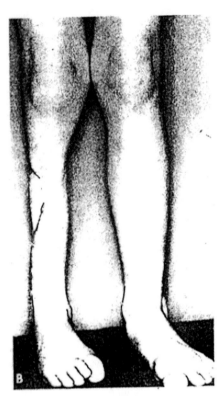

Figure 10-1. Leg with Compartment Syndrome

effect oxygen delivery within the ischemic bundle and keep some Na+ - K+ - ATP pumps running. Keep the patient well-hydrated. Remember he is losing fluid into the bundle and you need to keep perfusion pressures up. Also, those perfusion pressures are aided by keeping the limb level with the body. This will give you the best mean arterial pressure (MAP) without increasing intra-compartmental pressure and therefore give the best chance of flow.

Complications of compartment syndrome are permanent nerve damage (the ones that move your hands and feet), loss of the limb, cosmetic deformity, infection, and all its sequels down to SIRS, ARDS, and death on a ventilator. However, the quicker it is picked up, the better the prognosis. For patients who cannot feel, you need to rely on your neuro-vascular checks – warmth of the extremity, capillary refill, pulse, etc. One thing about pulse; by the time you have lost the pulse, you've probably lost the game. Losing the pulse is a very late sign of compartment syndrome. Unrelenting pain is your best sign. Remember that pain should be better every single day, and if it isn't, that's not normal. Suspect compartment syndrome.

In the picture on page 161, we see a patient who has had a good outcome from compartment syndrome, but look at the right leg. Would you like that leg? Muscle bundles are forever gone, making this leg permanently weaker than the other. There is terrible scarring with what appears to be skin grafts filling in between. And look at the foot -- this patient has foot drop. What a mess.

We tend to assume that our patients don't have compartment syndrome. They really have to scream and carry on a lot to get our attention. Because compartment syndrome is so devastating, please, for all you patients who could potentially have it, assume that they *do* have it. Make them prove to you that they don't have it. But if you ever have even the least little inkling that a patient might have compartment syndrome, get the cast cut off *immediately* and call a doctor.

Key Components in Chapter 10

1. Any time blood flow has been interrupted into a fascia bundle and started up again, the compartment is at risk for compartment syndrome.
2. The two pathways into increasing the pressure in the compartment to greater than the perfusion pressure are to
   a. Primarily raise the pressure in the compartment
   b. Shrink down the size of the compartment
3. The first sign of compartment syndrome is unrelenting pain. You should be able to medicate all post-op or trauma pain to a tolerable level, and if you can't, be highly suspicious that you might be looking at compartment syndrome.

Chapter 11

GI Emergencies

GI emergencies come in three kinds: 1) hemorrhage, 2) mechanical obstruction causing ischemia, and 3) ischemia from venous and arterial constriction secondary to systemic shock. When you die, one hundred percent of the time you die from a lethal dysrythmia. So, how can a GI bleed cause a lethal dysrythmia? Easy. Remember the four things that must be balanced to keep the heart beating are:

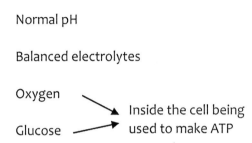

So, here is what happens with a GI emergency:

▼ volume ▶▼ oxygen delivery ▶ anaerobic metabolism ▶ lactic acid ▶ change in pH also;

▼ diastolic blood pressure ▶▼ oxygen into the heart ▶▼ ATP to repolarize the action potential ▶ lethal dysrythmia

There is less volume for circulation, so less oxygen is delivered to the cells. The cells go anaerobic, stop functioning properly, and begin cranking out lactic acid. Enough lactic acid changes the pH from normal to a metabolic acidosis, and that is one pathway into the lethal dysrythmia. Also, less oxygen is delivered into the heart because diastolic pressure has dropped (the force pushing the blood down the coronary arteries), it can't make enough ATP to repolarize the action potential, and that is another pathway into a lethal dysrythmia. As you well know, someone having a GI emergency can die very quickly.

In the same way that plaque builds up in your heart, carotids, or legs, it can also build up in the mesenteric arteries. If this happens, flow decreases as does ATP production, function, and infrastructure repair. You can infarct the gut just like you can infarct anything else. If you don't take care of infrastructure repair you can perforate the gut – big or small – which can make you very septic, leading to SIRS, leading to ARDS, leading to death on a ventilator. You can destroy your liver, causing death from hepatic failure with all that it entails.

You can also aspirate and have a terrible electrolyte imbalance from a GI obstruction. *Aspirate? Aspirate what? These patients aren't eating, what could they aspirate?* You and I produce eight liters of digestive fluids a day. We use it to digest our foods. It is very rich in electrolytes used to make hydrochloric acid, bicarb, and pancreatic enzymes. As we digest our food and things move on through the gut, the water and electrolytes are picked up and recycled into the body. The problem occurs when an obstruction of some type keeps things from flowing on through. You continue making the digestive enzymes, but they don't make it down to the pickup point, and the volume builds up like water behind a dam. This is what the patient aspirates and where the deficit in fluid and electrolytes occurs. Remember, you don't have to actually be eating food to generate digestive juices – all you need to do is to *think* about it.

You can also have an ischemic gut from the vasoconstriction caused by systemic shock. This is a good time to look at the effects of shock. First, let's look at the cellular effects of shock. On a cellular level, what is occurring when insufficient oxygen is delivered to the cell?

The Cellular Effects of Shock

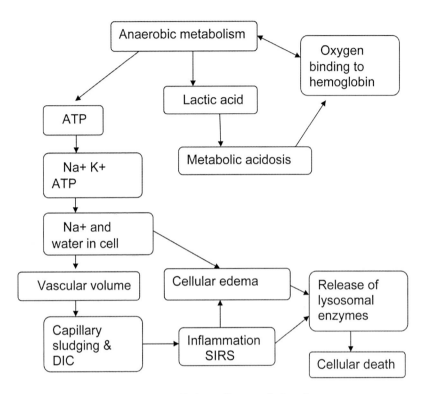

Figure 11-1. Cellular Effects of Shock

One definition of shock is that insufficient oxygen was delivered to the cell to maintain aerobic metabolism. Because of this, the functions of the cell cannot be maintained, and the cell also begins to make lactic acid. Enough lactic acid in the system causes a metabolic acidosis to develop. As I said earlier, being alkalotic will cause the red blood cell to hang on to oxygen at a cellular level, but being acidic will keep oxygen from attaching to the hemoglobin in the first place. Acidosis decreases the affinity of oxygen for hemoglobin, making our problem worse.

Now that the metabolism is anaerobic, there is insufficient ATP being generated, and the Na^+ - K^+ - ATP are not working well. The cell begins to swell up with water, causing cellular edema and dysfunction. If this goes on long enough, the swelling will begin to pull lysosomal membranes apart releasing caustic enzymes into the cell, which will produce cellular death. Enough dead cells and you get a dead human being.

Also, because there is so much of the body's water in the cells, there is a decrease in circulating volume. This decrease in volume causes changes in capillary flow via the pre- and post-capillary sphincters. The patient develops capillary sludging and goes into DIC. DIC is the hematological component of SIRS, setting off the inflammatory process throughout the body, causing more destruction of lysosomal membranes, and thereby cellular death. This is what happens in every cell in the body when insufficient oxygen is delivered to meet the cells' metabolic needs.

GI Bleeds

The problem with GI bleeds is that they cause you to lose perfusion volume and oxygen-carrying capacity. When making red blood cells – or anything else – problems of deficiency can have one of three causes: there is insufficient raw material available for building, the factory is not working right, or you are having a loss of the manufactured product.

Raw Material + Factory efficiency – Loss = Available supply

Deficiencies in the supply of raw material (biological substrates) needed for manufacturing can occur because it was not eaten, absorbed in the gut, or transported to the factory. Problems in the manufacturing of substances can come from assembly lines producing too much, too little, or an inferior quality of the desired substance. Supply is also determined by how much of the product is being lost from or destroyed by the body. Some early artificial heart valves are known to chew up red blood cells and chronic GI bleeds will cause them to be lost from the body.

Chronic GI bleeds are frequently detected because the patient develops an iron deficiency anemia. You recycle all of the iron used in your body to make red blood cells. When your body makes a new red blood cell, it lasts about 120 days. When it gets old and ratty, you tear it up and recycle 100% of the iron back into the bone marrow to make new red blood cells with. If a person develops an iron deficiency anemia, one easy way to make that happen is to have the red blood cells fall out of the body before the iron can be recycled. A slow, chronic GI bleed will do this nicely.

Let's look next at every nurse's favorite – the massive GI bleed.

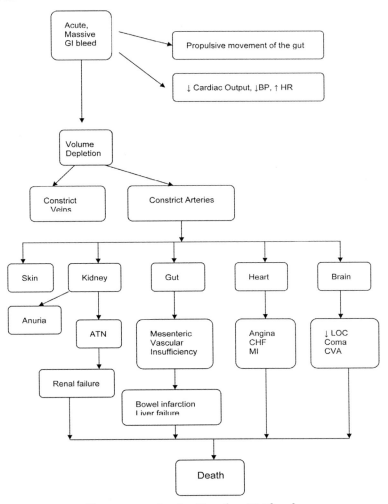

Figure 11-2. Acute Massive GI Bleed

Suppose a patient has just had a massive GI bleed. One of the first things you get is a propulsive movement of the gut, causing diarrhea. The effect of this is that the body doesn't have to metabolize all of that protein; the nurse can clean it up. The body considers this a plus. You may not.

The patient is now volume-depleted. This triggers venous and arterial vasoconstriction. The venous constriction has the effect of increasing blood volume and the arterial constriction increases perfusion pressures to help keep the blood circulating to vital areas. When you vasoconstrict into the skin, it becomes cold, clammy, and diaphoretic. Vasoconstrict into the kidneys and you stop making urine. If you do not keep your kidneys flushed, they clog up with debris, causing acute tubular necrosis, renal failure, and death. Decreasing blood flow into the gut decreases function, repair, and peristalsis. You can infarct the mesenteric arteries and/ or perforate the gut causing sepsis and SIRS, destroy or infarct the liver, and be dead from that.

Decreased blood flow into the heart is called myocardial ischemia. If you are inclined to feel it, it is called angina. The effect of it is decreased contractility leading to congestive heart failure, and you can have an MI. Also, with your change in level of consciousness, you can have a stroke. The question becomes, *"How in the world can you have an MI or a stroke from a hypovolemic event?"* Easy.

Let's say a person has some plaque in their carotid or left anterior descending artery in the heart. It may not be causing them much problem, it may be at critical mass, or anything in between these two extremes.

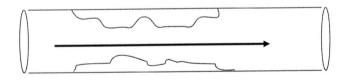

Everything is just fine until the hypovolemic episode, when the blood flow is either cut off or so severely restricted that flow slows down, the vessel walls come closer together, and a clot forms, completing the MI or CVA.

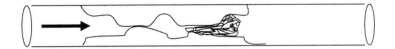

The way you would prevent this from happening is to keep the walls of the blood vessel pushed apart. What could you use to do this? Fluid. Lots and lots of fluid and nitrates. Preferably, you should use normal saline as it stays within the vessel better than some of the others. Blood products should be used as needed, because they are very good at not only adding oxygen-carrying capacity, but also at increasing the oncotic pressure within the blood vessel.

It is the oncotic pressure that draws fluid back into the blood vessels and keeps it from all leaking out of the circulatory system. Our blood vessels are semi-permeable, not lead pipes. Because you open and close slit pores, and because the pressure in the blood vessel is higher than that in the fluid surrounding the cells, volume always want to move from inside the blood vessel to outside. This isn't conducive to circulation and delivery to the cells. So, we combat the pressure to drive fluid out of the blood vessel with an equal pressure to pull it back into the blood vessel – the oncotic pressure.

The oncotic pressure is similar to osmosis. In school we all did an experiment where two fluids were separated by a semi-permeable membrane. One solution had lots of solutes in it and the other had none. We set up the experiment and went home. The next morning we found that the solution with lots of solutes had drawn water to it increasing its volume, but that now both solutions had the same amount of solutes. We called this osmosis. Oncotic pressure is the same, except we will use plasma proteins to make the gradient and pull fluid back into the blood vessel. Red blood cells make up a lot of the things in the blood made of protein. Other things that contribute to oncotic pressure are other blood cells, albumin, fibrinogen, etc. Having a normal hematocrit is about volume, oxygen-carrying capacity, and oncotic pressure. Without these things, we cannot oxygenate and perfuse at the same time.

Key Components in Chapter 11

1. Presence of a substance in the body depends on the availability of biological substrates with which to construct it, a functioning system of manufacture, and whether or not it is being lost from or destroyed in the body.

2. The problem with GI bleeds is that they cause death by lethal dysrhythmia, because the patient cannot oxygenate and or perfuse due to loss of volume and oxygen-carrying capacity and they interfere with the reabsorption of electrolytes from the GI tract.

3. Oncotic pressure is the force that draws fluid back into the blood vessel and it is made of plasma proteins.

Chapter 12

Conveying Your Concerns

Conveying your concerns to others requires a logical approach with precise language. These are statements written into patients' charts by people who were formerly thought to be intelligent.

The patient has chest pain if she lies on her side for over a year.

On the second day the knee was better, on the third day it disappeared.

She felt no rigors or shaking chills, but her husband states she was hot in bed last night.

The patient is tearful and crying constantly. She also appears to be depressed.

The patient has been depressed since she began seeing me in 1993.

Discharge status: alive, but without permission.

Healthy appearing, decrepit 69 year old male, mentally alert but forgetful.

The patient refused autopsy.

The patient had no previous history of suicide.

The patient has left white blood cells at another hospital.

The patient's medical history has been remarkably insignificant with only a 40 pound weight gain in the last three days.

The patient had waffles for breakfast and anorexia for lunch.

Between you and me, we ought to be able to get this lady pregnant.

Since she can't get pregnant with her husband, I thought you might like to work her up.

She is numb from her toes down.

While in the ER, she was examined, x-rated, and sent home.

The skin was moist and dry.

Occasional, constant, infrequent headaches.

Patient alert and unresponsive.

Rectal examination revealed a normal size thyroid.

She stated that she had been constipated most of her life until she got a divorce.

Both breasts were equal and reactive to light and accommodation.

Examination of the genitalia reveals that he is circus sized.

The patient was to have a bowel resection; however, he took a job as a stockbroker instead.

Skin: somewhat pale but present.

The pelvic exam will be done later on the floor.

The patient was seen in consultation by Dr. Smith, who felt we should sit on the abdomen, and I agree.

Large brown stool ambulating in the hall.

The patient has two teenage children, but no other abnormalities.

When she fainted her eyes rolled around the room.

MD at bedside attempting to urinate times three.

Vaginal packing out. Doctor in.

Patient was in his usual good health until his plane ran out of gas and crashed.

Getting Others to See Through Your Eyes

You have been a very diligent observer and now need to convey your concerns to other people. How do you get them to pay attention and see what you see? You must paint a vivid picture, whether you are charting or doing a verbal report. You must be organized in stating your case – everything in chronological order with complete vital signs and lab data. No skipping around, no late entries. The questions that need answering are who, what, when, where, what did you do, effect, what are you doing now, who did you tell, what did they say – just like they told us in nursing school.

Most of us use computerized charting today. In the good old days, when we wrote out our nurse's notes by longhand, we wrote a lot of silly things trying to fill up space. We also wrote very important things about our perception of the problem. Today with electronic charting, you may have the options of "black" or "white" when what you really wanted to say was "gray." You still need to say "gray." In your electronic charting, it may come under comments, nurse's notes, or one group wrote in longhand in the physician's progress pages if something untoward had happened to their patient.

From time to time, lawyers send me patients' charts for me to review looking to see if the nurse followed the nursing standard of care. The nursing standard of care is, 1) did you perceive the problem, 2) did you tell the doctor, and 3) if you didn't get a satisfactory answer from the doctor, did you go up the chain of command to get a good outcome for your patient?

Lawyers know you don't have any money. They are after your hospital's malpractice fund, which should have lots of money. If the family sues the doctor and you did not go up the chain of command, you get to sit right next to him all the way through his malpractice trial (and you may not like him well enough to have to do this).

One beautiful side effect of the Rapid Response Team is that calling them qualifies as going up the chain of command. Get other people involved. Don't just chart and wring your hands – you are legally obligated to go up the chain of command. It is not an option!

Sometime the doctors are very tuned into what we are trying to tell them, but we just throw a bunch of numbers at them. Two patients can have exactly the same vital signs. One is getting better with them; the other is dying with them. You have to give the doctor some clues. You are looking at this in 3D living color, with sight, smells, and tension in the air – but the doctor gets little trickles of grey on the phone.

Here is a patient on the post-op floor so incredibly fluid overloaded that she has pink foam coming out of her mouth. The nurse calls the surgeon and says, "Her pressure is dropping." What did the surgeon order? Fluids, of course, because the surgeon knows about the response to injury and increased capillary permeability. The nurse gave the patient a liter of fluid because the doctor ordered it, and of course the patient died. Apparently, pink foam coming out of the patient's mouth did not mean pulmonary edema to this nurse, but I bet if she would have described the patient to the doctor, it would have meant everything to the surgeon. You don't have to know what to call something; you just need to describe it. Get the doctor to see through your eyes.

What Did You Do and What Effect Did It Have

What did you do about it and what effect did it have? We are usually good at explaining what we did, but we tend to neglect explaining the effect of our actions. You gave the patient a nitroglycerine tablet for his chest pain? That's nice. How is he? Dead on the floor, or sitting in the chair reading a book? You accidentally dc'd his epidural catheter, so you started him on oral pain medication. That's nice. How is he? Writhing in pain, or watching the football game on TV?

What Are You Doing Now

What are you doing now? When you sign off from your charting, it looks as if you never went into the patient's room again. Actually, you were in there a lot. You hung a new antibiotic, the doctor came by, RT gave a nebulizer treatment that you'd ordered – it was a busy place. But when someone else looks at the chart, it seems as if you said, *"Well, my shift is over. I hope he lives until they get out of report."* When you sign off from your charting, always say what you are continuing to do about the problem so that it shows your continued presence and attention to the patient.

Vital Information to Include
- Diaphoretic
- Work effort
- Fatigability
- Patient's body position
- Is the patient passing the look test?
- Patient says this is the "worst ever"
- Patient says this is "different from previous episodes"
- Any signs of poor cardiac output
- Any signs of compartment syndrome
- New onset heart murmur

Paint the picture for the doctor boldly so he can see through your eyes. Is the patient diaphoretic? We now know that is a very ominous sign signifying maximal sympathetic stimulation. How hard is the patient working to achieve those numbers? How long do you think he can keep it up? Fatigability can cause a sudden deterioration in a patient's condition.

What is the patient's body position? Is he lying flat in bed? Does he have the head of the bed up 30 degrees? Or is he like a patient I had one time who had pulled a chair over to the sink, put a pillow across the sink, and was trying to sleep with severe pulmonary edema. The patient's body position will tell you how stressed they are with those numbers.

If the patient has had this occur to him before, is this event the same as past ones? More or less severe? Episodes that are the "worst ever" or "different from previous episodes" require a doctor. Is the patient passing the "Look Test?" – how does the patient look to you? Is the patient exhibiting any of the signs of poor cardiac output that were discussed earlier?

- Change in level of consciousness
- Respiratory distress anywhere on the continuum
- Heart rate up
- Liver down
- GI problems increased
- Urine output decreased
- Exercise capacity has dropped off

Is the girth increased or the amount of edema changing? This is more difficult to assess in the post-op patient because all post-op patients are edematous secondary to the capillary slit pores opening in response to injury. Does the patient have any signs of compartment syndrome? Does the patient have a new onset heart murmur? How do you find out if he had the murmur yesterday? The easiest and most accurate way to find out is to look in the "Impression" section of the doctor's H&P. This is where the doctor lays it out clear as a bell as to what is wrong with this patient.

Aortic stenosis
1. Atrial fibrillation
2. Coumadin therapy
3. Type II diabetes, etc, etc, etc

This information is worth its weight in gold and it belongs on the patients Kardex (or whatever it is called at your institution) in the history section. Our patients complain over and over that we think we can come into their rooms and take care of them and we don't have a clue who they are. You might get away with it for a while, but the day will come when you will make a big mistake because you didn't know the patient's history. Our patients are sicker than ever before and our care must be more comprehensive than ever before.

An elderly lady had colon cancer and needed a colectomy. She also had a bad heart. The surgeon sent her to a cardiologist and said, *"Do your best."* The cardiologist took her off to the cath lab and angioplastied open several of her coronary arteries, started her on cardiac drugs, stabilized her, and sent her back to the surgeon saying, *"Good luck."* She did very well post-op. She began to drink on time, eat on time, and was due to go home the next day when she crashed and burned during the middle of the night.

Her cardiac meds had never beet restarted post-op. The history section on her Kardex was blank. None of the nurses taking care of her had any idea that she had had an angioplasty two weeks previous. Was it important for them to know? You bet it was, and by not knowing they greatly compromised this patient's care. *"But, wait,"* you might say. *"It's not my job to start the meds back up!"* Have you figured out what your job as a nurse is yet? You are the great coordinator and suggester. It is the nurse that says to the doctor *"Is it time to ...?"* Or *"Would you like to ...?"* When the nurse doesn't know the patient's history, care suffers.

What is caring, anyway? What does it mean to care? The best definition I ever heard for the word caring came from Holocaust survivor Elie Wiesel in his book Night. He said caring was having a willingness to intervene. If you care if your patient goes home again, one of the most powerful things you can do is to get the patient's history from the impression section of the H&P, put it on the patient's Kardex, and incorporate it into your spiel for report. Your spiel goes something like, *"Down in room 234 is Mr. Smith, who is a 67-year-old patient of Dr. Smith in with a thoracotomy, **and who has a history of blah, blah, blah.**"* This way, everyone sitting in report hears that the patient only has one kidney, or hears that this man has already had two sets of heart bypass grafts, or hears that this surgery was done for cancer. If you do this, you will greatly enhance the patient's care and increase his chances for survival.

Key Concepts in Chapter 12

1. Use descriptives, not just numbers, to convey your concerns. Get the doctors to see through your eyes. They aren't mind readers.
2. You are legally obligated to go up the chain of command if you aren't satisfied with a doctor's answer. It is not an option; you have to.
3. Know your patient's history!

Chapter 13

How We Learn

Knowledge is essential to critical thinking and to progressing through the stages of proficiency, so let's spend some time looking at the latest information about how we learn.

We used to teach that memory was both short- and long-term and that it was like a series of filing cabinets that opened and closed based on need. It turns out to be a much more elaborate operation. Because of modern technological advances, we are now able to view the changes which occur in brain activity as we think and learn. Computerized tomography (CT scan) is excellent at looking at structures, but cannot determine functioning in the brain. Because we know that the only energy source in the body is ATP (made of oxygen plus glucose), increased functioning will require an increase in ATP in that area of the brain. Therefore, if we can follow ATP, we should be able to follow brain function. There are two ways to accomplish this.

One is to follow glucose, since it is a key ingredient in ATP formation. Positron emission tomography studies (PET scans) follow radioactively tagged glucose to see where it is used in the brain. Active sites "light up" when more of the radioactive glucose is used. PET scans show shifts and changes in brain activity along with changes in mental and physical activity. Using PET scans allows researchers to see what parts of the brain are active in learning and memory.

Magnetic resonance imaging (MRI scans) offers clear and precise looks at the body's internal structure. Because the MRI takes pictures so fast, it is able to record changes that occur once a second. But that is still a structural look, not a look at how the body functions.

Glucose and oxygen are delivered to the cells to make ATP via the circulatory system. This is not a set flow, as it differs based on the needs of the tissue. More active tissue will need a greater blood flow to deliver more of the building blocks required for the

ATP to meet the increased need. If you were able to follow blood flow precisely and very rapidly, an image of the brain at work would become clear. Functional MRIs (fMRI) scans do precisely this by using very rapid pictures of structures overlaid with circulatory patterns. You can generate moving pictures of brain activity as a person responds to stimuli, acts, or, in our area of interest, learns.

This new technology allows scientists to see the changes that go on in the human brain as we learn. Neuroplasticity is the term used for the brain's ability to continually reorganize itself based on new information. This continues throughout our lifetime, but is especially rapid during childhood. We learn throughout our lifetimes, but we do it in different ways once we become adults.

Basic Brain Facts

Your brain weighs a little over three pounds and if you mess with it too much, it will fall apart. It is grapefruit-sized, walnut shaped, and would lay comfortably in the palm of your hand. The brain represents two percent of our body weight, but consumes 20% of our daily calories. ATP = glucose + oxygen. Glucose = calories. Twenty percent of our daily calories equals a lot of action.

Eighty percent of the brain by weight is the cerebrum. Its two hemispheres are connected by the 200 million bi-directional nerve fibers which make up the *corpus callosum*. The surface, or cortex (tree bark), is only 1/10 of an inch thick (or the width of three hairs) and contains only six layers of cells. Because of its surface convolutions there are 2.5 square feet of surface area. In each cubic inch there are 10,000 miles of connection fibers. It is within the cortex that thinking, memory, speech, and muscle movement occur.

The Gender Differences in Brain Structure
- ♂ have a higher % of gray matter in the left hemisphere than ♀. In ♀ it is the same in both hemispheres.
- ♂ have more neurons in the cerebral cortex; ♀ have more connections between the neurons.

- ♂ & ♀ language areas are in the left hemisphere. ♀ also have an active language center in the right hemisphere.
- When recalling emotions, ♀ use a larger portion of their limbic system than do ♂. ♀ are better at recognizing different types of emotions in other people.

The frontal lobe of the brain acts as a type of executive control center which monitors higher order thinking and directs problem solving. It also modulates the excesses of the emotional system. This area is where you tell yourself to calm down and think – everything will work out. This is also where self-will and personality occur. This portion of the brain is not fully operational in adolescence!

The cerebellum has long been known to control muscle coordination, but it also appears to be important in learning, performance, and the timing of complex motor tasks. This is where we store rote memory like how to tie a shoelace or ride a bike. New research has shown that it might also help us fine tune our thoughts and emotions as well as play a part in recalling memories.

Only one-tenth of the composition of the cerebral cortex is composed of neurons. The remaining 90% is made of glial (glue) cells that hold the neurons together, filter out harmful substances, and regulate the rate of neuron signaling. There are, nevertheless, 100 billion neurons in the brain capable of carrying 250 to 2,500 impulses per second.

Each neuron is capable of having tens of thousands of dendrites (trees) projecting from its body. Because of that, there are one quadrillion possible synaptic junctions that can be used for learning and storage of events. Because of this huge number of possible junctions, each individual human being has his own unique pattern of connections. This is why no two of us see the world in the exact same way, or recall the same events in precisely the same way.

Unlike the dendrites, each neuron has only one axon (axis). The axon is surrounded by the myelin sheath that insulates and speeds up the impulse traveling the axon. Impulses travel from the axon to the dendrite of connecting cells via synaptic (joining together) junctions utilizing neurotransmitters. Acetylcholine, epinephrine, serotonin and dopamine are well known examples of neurotransmitters, but there are actually over 100 neurotransmitters known to scientists today. Learning causes changes in the synapses and thereby the effect of one neuron upon another.

The brain has two hemispheres joined together by the corpus callosum. The two hemispheres have different functions. The left is responsible for analysis, sequences, and speech, and recognizes words, letters and numbers. The function of the left hemisphere is to process time-sensitive input sequentially. Spoken language is found on the left side as is the ability to do math problems. It is the left side of the brain that seeks explanations for events.

The right hemisphere, however, is more creative, sees patterns in current and past activities, is more concerned with where things are in space and with situational context. This side interprets language through gestures and facial movement and likes to place events in spatial patterns.

The right hemisphere is very different from the left hemisphere, but it is very important that they talk to each other to get the "whole picture". It is the corpus callosum that provides the communication pathway. Its pathways are bi-directional and allow each hemisphere to utilize the information and resources of the other.

Should the corpus callosum be severed, as is sometimes done to control seizures, interesting things begin to happen. When researchers cover the right eye of such a patient and teach the left eye to recognize pictures when the left eye is covered, the exposed right eye cannot recognize the pictures the left eye had seen because there was no communication between the hemispheres.

The two halves of the brain have independent capabilities for consciousness, memory storage, communication, and control of motor activities. The corpus callosum is required for the two sides to operate cooperatively . . . [it] plays an additional role in unifying the emotional responses of the brain. (Guyton, 10th edition, p. 671)

Emotions play a huge part in learning. If an event does not cause a significant reward or punishment, we barely remember it. Ninety-nine percent of the stimuli that enters our brain falls in this category. It is perceived, found not to make us happy or sad, and is quickly forgotten. There are separate centers in the brain for reward and punishment and stimulating one or the other causes learning. Repeated stimulation of the punishment center can render the pleasure center nonfunctional. If too many bad things happen to a person, it becomes very hard to find pleasure in anything. We will look later at the effect of punishment on learning in the clinical environment.

Learning and the Limbic System

The limbic (border) system controls emotions and motivational drive. Emotions, as I have said, play a large part in learning, and it is what we have learned that gives us our motivation and behavior. The parts of the limbic system that deal with memory and learning are the *hypothalamus*, *hippocampus* (seahorse), and *amygdala* (almond).

The hypothalamus plays a central part in the limbic system, but also regulates the autonomic nervous system and the secretion of hormones from both the anterior and posterior pituitary glands. The hypothalamus controls the reward and punishment centers for the limbic system. If we are punished, we tend to withdraw unless the stimulus is very strong – then it can produce a response of rage. On the other hand, rewards make us docile. In this way, the hypothalamus controls what we choose to learn or ignore. People will participate in learning activities that have been successful, while avoiding those that have produced failure (Sousa, 2001).

The hippocampus is important in recalling events from stored memory into working memory. We recall past events and compare them to current events for pattern recognition.

Recognizing patterns and similarities to past events is a large component of intuition and critical thinking. This area of the brain also consolidates and converts memory from short-term to long-term for storage.

The amygdala (almond) is part of the limbic system, and operates in a semi-conscious state while transmitting information regarding both surroundings and thoughts. It is believed to govern behavior appropriate to the situation. It has abundant bi-directional connections with the other parts of the limbic system and the rest of the brain, and it has been called the window through which the brain sees a person's place in the world. Should there be a bilateral ablation of the amygdala, test animals develop Klüver-Bucy syndrome. Symptoms include a lack of fear, extreme curiosity about everything, forgetting rapidly, having a tendency to place objects in the mouth, trying to eat solid objects, and an extremely strong sex drive.

Types of Memory

What is a memory? Memories are caused by changes that occur in synaptic junctions that are caused by neural activity. Neural pathways (memory traces) are laid down to help facilitate recall. Actual physiological changes occur when learning takes place, in order to establish these memory traces. The more often the memory is used, the stronger the pathway becomes.

Different kinds of memory include skilled, semantic, episodic, and productive. Skilled memory occurs because of strong neural pathways generated by frequent retrieval. This is also called expertise. We store diagnostic concepts, theories, and knowledge in our semantic memory. Our episodic memory includes our personal experiences and tells us what to do if various events arise – if *this*, then you do *that*. Productive memory is a blend of episodic and semantic that increases with experience and is lacking in novices due to their complete lack of experiences.

In the past, I taught my students that there was short-term and long-term memory, and that activating a memory was similar to going to a filing cabinet, opening the right drawer, and pulling the right file. Well it is, but it is also much more than that. Using new technology, researchers have discovered that memories are not stored in one spot but are, rather, all over the brain. For recall to occur, the different sites must be activated to reconstruct the memory in what are called convergence zones. When you think of a fresh orange many things come to mind. There is the feel of the orange in your hand, the color, texture, smell, taste, whether you like or dislike them, good and bad experiences you have had around oranges, etc. We now think that the component parts of "orange" are stored in different parts of the brain and must be all pulled back together to generate your memory of a fresh orange. This is much more complex than we had originally thought.

We still recognize short-term memory, but we now believe it has two component parts. In *immediate memory*, data is held for about 30 seconds while it is determined whether or not it is of immediate importance to us. The siren in the distance; is it coming toward us or going away? Do we need to respond? Our past experience plays heavily here. What do we know about sirens in the distance? If the stimulus is deemed not to be important, it is dropped from the system immediately.

The next form of short-term memory is *working memory*, where there is conscious processing of current and past data -- and where learning takes place. Unfortunately, it has limited capacity. Most people can hold only five to nine (7 plus or minus 2) pieces of information at a time. Too many tasks or too much input can cause a meltdown in a novice. Remember, for a lot of us, remembering five things at once really taxes the system. You need to see how your learner is doing before pushing on with more information. Goleman's (1995) *Emotional Intelligence* tells us that how a person "feels" about a situation determines how much time and effort will be put into learning.

Data that affects survival and/or generates strong emotions are processed first. This has a tremendous impact on people orienting to a new job. Fear and trepidation slow learning,

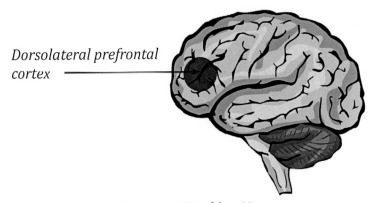

Dorsolateral prefrontal cortex

Figure 13-1. Working Memory

and orienting to new job is a very scary thing. So much is riding on your success; the house or car payment, stability at home, your self-esteem. If I fail does it mean a move for the kids, do we lose the house, do I end up back on the night shift in the job I just left behind? Preceptors must do much to alleviate this anxiety. The novice must understand that you have a commitment to training and retaining new hires. There are proficiencies that must be passed, but they are not the end of the world. The more threatened your new hires are, the less likely they are to ask questions.

The learner must feel "physically safe and emotionally secure" (Sousa, 2001) for learning to take place. Learners with emotional or physical problems taking up their time and energy will do poorly in learning situations. It is better to let them go and take care of their problems that to try to continue teaching them.

Because short-term memory is so limited in size, and because we frequently need to consider more than 9 things at once, we have a method for consolidating material called chunking. In *chunking*, we perceive a set of data as a single item. Sets of letters become words, 4915082627 becomes (491) 508-2627. In this manner we can hold much more information in our short-term memory because we make discernable patterns. In the phrase *"grandma is buying an apple,"* 22 letters become 5 chunks. We add visual images based on our past experience of old ladies buying apples.

LSDN BCT VF BIU SA is difficult to make sense out of because we have no past memory of these groupings of letters. LSD NBC TV FBI and USA are much easier to remember because they are connected to past events. Assigning meaning based on past events is called *coding*. We need to speak to new learners in a language they understand. With an experienced ICU nurse, it is appropriate to talk about stroke volume in relation to cardiac function. For the novice, it is more appropriate to talk about the amount of water that comes out each time you push down on the handle of an old fashioned hand-crank pump when describing stroke volume. Talk in a language your learner understands. You will eventually work your way up to scientific terms and concepts.

For learning to take place, data must be stored in long-term memory. Distinctive physiological changes take place in the brain when learning takes place. In the following PET scan, the difference between practiced and unpracticed skills is glaringly obvious.

UNPRACTICED

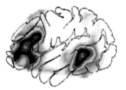

PRACTICED

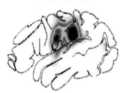

Figure 13-2. PET scan

Physiological changes that take place in the neuron are detailed by Guyton in his *Textbook of Medical Physiology*. As the number of sites that release the neurotransmitter at the synapse increase and more of the neurotransmitter is made, the number of synaptic terminals for receiving the neurotransmitter can as much as double. This will cause the dendrite that the connection is for to enlarge and transmit stronger signals, and learning occurs. Fifty percent of the neural connections we are born with are eliminated over time because we don't use them. Our brain is a *"use it or lose it"* system.

In order for working memory to go into long-term, the data must be consolidated. This requires codification with similar memories so that effective recall can occur. This takes time – 5 minutes for minimal and 1 hour for strong consolidation. If anything interrupts the process, like strong emotion, consolidation may not occur and the learning can be lost.

It is the hippocampus that promotes the storage of memories. Patients who have had the hippocampi removed for treatment of epilepsy are unable to store new memories. They remember perfectly the data stored in their brain before the surgery, but are incapable of remembering new verbal or symbolic data for more than a few minutes. A possible explanation is that the hippocampus is dominant as an input pathway to the reward and punishment areas of the limbic system. Without these pathways, new data becomes emotionally neutral, is considered unimportant, and ends up dumped from the system.

Data is stored in long-term memory so we can remember it. Remembering is a conscious process that takes the old, stored memory apart and updates it with new information. When this mixture of old and new data is sent back into long-term memory, new proteins are made to hold the new structure. It is not the same as it was before.

What is the probability of storage in long-term memory? The best learning takes place when you have a need to know. Adult learners learn best if you take an event that is familiar to them and then add a new fact – adults learn very quickly this way. The data also has to have relevance to their current lives for them to expend the energy to learn. Who wants to take a course in bicycle maintenance

if they don't own a bicycle? But if you are going on a biking tour of the Netherlands where you are responsible for maintaining your own bike, it then becomes very relevant and you will be eager to learn.

The hippocampus encodes the information and sends it off to one or more storage areas. The actual storage occurs during deep sleep. That's right; at night. How much good sleep you get determines how much you will have learned from the day's teachings. What this means is that if you don't get enough sleep, you can't learn. Most of us need eight to nine hours of sleep – some of us 10 to 12 hours. It varies from person to person.

Storage in long-term memory is also facilitated by carbohydrate intake. It takes glucose to make ATP, which means you need to eat. How many times have nurses worked a shift straight through without a meal? The brain can only use glucose to make ATP. Other organs in the body can use other sources, but not the brain – it is glucose driven. If you do not eat, you do not think and learn as effectively. Make sure your learner eats, otherwise all he will remember from the shift is how tired he was.

To retain what you have learned, you must repeat it. Do it again, and again, and again. Before a skill is truly learned, it must be repeated seven times. Seven times! We usually give the learner one or two tries, but *true learning requires seven successful completions of the task.* We learn best when we are given positive reinforcement.

Types of Intelligence

Intelligence is a multifaceted aptitude that varies even within the same individual. It can be defined as simply the rate of learning something.

Sousa, 2001

In the past we were taught that there is only one type of intelligence – the kind that is measured on standardized IQ tests. Today, we know there are many kinds of intelligence, which are *not* reflected on IQ tests. None of us are all one or the other type of intelligence, but rather a blend of them all with a preference for one or two. Humans are too complex to describe in just a few words, but we continue to try and do it anyway with our classification systems. When looking at an oversimplified classification system, we need to remember that no one is all this factor or all that factor. We have all the traits in us to a degree, but we do have one or two that we prefer most.

There are numerous authors who describe different kinds of intelligence with varying numbers of categories. They all have their pros and cons; here are some examples:

Linguistic
Do you consider yourself good with words and their meanings?
Can you explain things simply and concisely when necessary?
Can you remember things you have read and heard?
This form of intelligence is all about how we deal with language, words and their meanings and is often highly developed in writers and poets.

Logical-Mathematical
- Are you good at solving problems?
- Do you find it easy to work with numbers?
- Do you sit watching illusionists on TV and try and figure how they do it?

This form of intelligence relates to how we reason and solve problems and is often highly developed in mathematicians, scientists, engineers, and computer programmers.

Spatial
- If someone describes the layout of their house to you, do you find it easy to visualize it your head?
- Can you imagine what your lounge would look like painted in green and orange polka dots?
- Are you good at judging distances?
- Can you tell which way is North?

This form of intelligence relates to how we visualize and perceive physical space in our heads and is often highly developed in chess players, architects and in home designers.

Musical
- Have you found it easy to learn to play an instrument?
- Can you sing in tune and tell when others aren't?
- Do you compose your own music?
- Do you have rhythm?
- Can you tell when someone playing an instrument has played a bad note?

This form of intelligence is not just about music and composition. It is also about our ability to identify pitches and rhythms from the sounds we hear around us everyday. As you would expect, this form of intelligence is often highly developed in professional musicians and DJ's, but also sound engineers, record producers and, in some cases, mechanics, who can diagnose a fault from the sound a car makes.

Bodily-Kinesthetic
- Do you consider yourself a skillful sports player?
- On the dance floor, do you believe you can dance, instead of being someone who randomly moves their arms and legs?
- Could you walk a tightrope, even if it was just a few centimeters off the ground?
- How easy do you find it to thread a needle?
- Can you pat your head while rubbing your stomach?

This form of intelligence relates to how skillful we are in the movement and use of our body and is often associated with professional athletes, dancers, and circus artists.

Naturalist
- Do you love being around animals?
- Can you identify different types of trees?
- Can you identify the different star constellations?
- Are flowers all the same to you?
- Have you ever tried to catch a snowflake to see what it looked like?

This intelligence involves the recognition of patterns and the classification of the natural world. It can be seen in astronomers, birdwatchers, and farmers.

Interpersonal
- Do you like meeting new people?
- Do you find it easy working with a team of people?
- Do you find that people often tell you their problems because you are a good listener or give good advice?
- Do you remain patient when trying to teach someone something you are good at or you know more about?

This form or intelligence is often highly developed in individuals whose work is people oriented, for instance, teachers, counselors, hairdressers and receptionists.

Intrapersonal
- Do you know what your strengths and weaknesses are?
- Do you allow yourself to show emotion?
- Would you describe yourself as spiritual?

This form of intelligence relates to an understanding of our private, innermost selves. You can probably think of people you know who probably wouldn't score highly on this at all – and others, who would.

Learning Styles
The point of putting these forms of intelligence into the book was to show that we all have multiple forms of intelligence and we learn in different ways. You need to match the preceptor,

his learning style, and his preference for learning to the novice at the very beginning of his orientation. This should give the greatest comfort all around and facilitate learning.

What is your preferred way of learning? First of all, are you an auditory or visual learner? Do you want to be told about procedures you are learning about, or read about them? Do you need to touch what you are trying to learn in order to understand new data? Keep in mind that, once again, we are mixture of types, but have preferences.

Take a minute and write your phone number in the space below.

Did you see it in front of you as you recalled it and read it to yourself or did you hear it spoken in your mind? Visual learners see it, auditory learners hear it. Do not mix a strongly-grounded visual learner with someone who wants to tell them how things are put together. Don't show an auditory person a lot of pictures because they want to hear you explain it. About 85% of us are visual, 15% are auditory, and a few of us can't learn anything unless we have something in our hand. I am very, very visual. Do not tell me what needs to be done; I can retain very little of what I am told. But at the same time, as I have matured, I have found that saying things out loud can help me remember – sometimes.

Keeping in mind that we are not all any one thing but a mixture of all the learning styles, knowing the teacher's and student's preferences can greatly facilitate learning. The worst orientation I ever had was to a cath lab. The teacher was incredibly auditory; there were no graphs, pictures, or models anywhere. He talked me through complex procedures and expected me to remember them the next day. I was frantic, because I am highly visual! The best orientation I ever had was to a newborn intensive care. I had a preceptor at my side for three months. There were books, illustrations, and movies all over the place. I was in heaven. I loved both jobs, once I got on my feet, but I hope to never orient with an auditory teacher again as long as I live. You need to match the student to the teacher for optimal learning to occur.

Key Components in Chapter 13

1. We have learned that, in order for learning to take place, the information must be relevant, in a language the learner can understand, presented at a rate the learner can assimilate, and be conducted in a non-threatening environment, and the learner must be fed and have had sufficient sleep. Repetition, repetition, repetition, and positive reinforcement in a happy work area. There must be a time to rest and a time to ask questions. Not too much to ask, is it?

2. There are many kinds of intelligence and different preferred ways of learning. Team teachers with similar learners.

Chapter 14

Critical Thinking Skills at Differing Levels of Nursing Proficiency

A novice nurse and an experienced nurse are involved in a clinical crisis. The experienced nurse steps in and takes care of the problem. After it is all over, the novice nurse turns to the experienced nurse and says, "*Why did you do that?*" The experienced nurse replies, "*That's what you are supposed to do.*" This makes the novice crazy, because she cannot mentally go from the patient care situation to "*That's what you're supposed to do.*" They cannot make the links, because they do not have the experience or the knowledge to make those links. The novice feels that she will never advance in nursing because it is just too complicated. Her anxiety level goes up, her learning goes down and the experienced nurse feels that the novice "*just doesn't get it.*"

You bring the two divergent sides together with knowledge, experience, and a tool – knowledge and experience because those are the requirements for critical thinking, and a tool so that both sides are speaking the same language. For the knowledge component we have the first chapters of this book. The tool for this presentation will be the Whiteside Critical Thinking Model. The understanding for the stages of proficiency in nursing practice will be those discussed in Benner's (1984, 2001) *From Novice to Expert*. By the novice, experienced nurse, and the manager understanding how we learn and the stages of proficiency, we should be able to assist and enhance learning and critical thinking in all our nurses.

When Critical Thinking is Absent

Sometimes it is easiest to understand the concept of critical thinking by seeing when it is absent. In 1854, Florence Nightingale went to nurse the British Army soldiers of the Crimean War. The conditions were atrocious and made worse by a complete lack of critical thinking on the part of those who were in charge. Things were so bad that the McNeill & Tulloch Commission was sent out from London to find out what the problem was. This is part of their report:

> Lime juice, though present, was not issued to the troops because there was no order for it to be dispensed on land; only when the troops were on board ship (McNeill & Tulloch, 1855, p. 8). There was a great need for a soft bread as opposed to hardtack. This was recognized by the Commissariat, and a floating bakery was being constructed in England and was due to arrive in several months. Meanwhile, no prevision was made to use the local bakeries (p. 9). Green coffee was issued for the troops to grind and roast themselves even though there were 2,705 pounds of tea in the Commissariat store in Balaclava (p. 9). Fresh coffee was available in Constantinople but there was no procedure for the Army to purchase it.
>
> The troops were expected to cook their own food and gather their own firewood. "For a time there was little difficulty in procuring firewood; but after the brushwood in the vicinity of the camp was consumed, fuel could not be obtained except by digging up roots, an operation which, to unskilled hands, involved great labour, and, in bad weather, much exposure" (McNeill & Tulloch, 1855, p. 10). The Commissariat said it could not help the situation because, "soldiers were not entitled to a ration of fuel unless in barracks." The Commissary had a fuel depot at Scutari, but would not issue it to the troops in the field (p. 10). The result, Russell (1856) says is, "That the food is often devoured in its raw state, or the tired soldier contented himself with merely rum and biscuit" (p. 19).

When supplies arrived, often they were not issued to those who needed them. McNeill and Tulloch (1855) found that of the 12,000 great-coats that arrived, 9000 remained in the stores while soldiers suffered frostbite from exposure to the icy winter. The reason the coats were not issued was that a soldier is allowed only one coat every three years, and few of the troops qualified for new coats (p. 27). Soldiers would be issued only what was included in their warrants and doctors could be punished for "setting aside the authority of the warrant" (p. 28).

We have all heard of the Charge of the Light Brigade and its lethal outcome, but few of us know what happened to the horses that survived.

Eight hundred tons of hay had been contracted to be sent to the Crimea, but the contractor was unable to meet order partially due to the lack of financial backing by the banks in London. Because of various causes, hay was never purchased in the Crimea for the horses. When talking about the horses used in the infamous Charge of the Light Brigade, McNeill and Tulloch state,

> The whole Brigade remained in this state until the 2nd of December, when it was directed to return to its previous position, but by that time the horses were reduced to such a state from starvation, that they could no longer bear the weight of their riders, they had to be led down; many were left on the ground in a dying state, and the remainder seventeen died on the road before they could reach their former station, a distance of only about six miles. (p. 20)

The horses starved to death because no one could think out of the box enough to buy hay from local farmers. The men couldn't have replacement coats because of a rule that did not allow for special circumstances and no one was willing to thwart the rules even though men were dying. That is, until Florence Nightingale arrived:

In 1855, the boiler in the laundry at the Barrack Hospital broke down and no official could be found that felt it was within his authorization to have it repaired, although all agreed that it needed to be. The result was that there were no laundry facilities at the hospital and therefore no clean clothes, linens, or blankets available to the thousands of patients. The official inaction caused Nightingale to purchase boilers from the Army Engineer's Office herself and establish a laundry house for the hospital (Dossey, 1999).

We want staff who can see what needs to be done and follow tasks through until proper completion. We have just seen what happens when there is no critical thinking. If we want critical thinkers, what is it we are asking for?

What is Critical Thinking?

The origins of critical thinking can be found with the ancient Greeks. The word "critical" is derived from the Greek *kritein*, which means to choose or decide. The Greek noun *krites* means judge; and the English word *criterion* meaning a standard, rule, or method also has a Greek derivation. Plato defined thinking as "the intercourse within" over 2,300 years ago (McKinzie, 1992).

There are as many definitions of critical thinking as there are authors of papers addressing the concept. In 1964, Watson and Glaser defined critical thinking as "being disposed to consider in a thoughtful way the problems and subjects that come within the range of one's experience" (cited in Beck et al, 1992, pg.5). It is this "being disposed" to think critically that has been difficult for a lot of nurses because they have been taught to follow doctor's orders rather than to think on their own.

Critical thinking is a voluntary action. A person must want to use any critical thinking skills that he may have (Norris, 1989). If someone is not predisposed to use these skills, there is no ascertainable benefit in having them. For example, the nurse may possess a high degree of critical thinking, but if s/he does not feel that the data are valued or important and should be reported, critical thinking most likely will not take place.

The second component of Watson and Glaser's definition of critical thinking reads "within the range of one's experience." I cannot think critically about what kind of steel to put into a bridge. I haven't a clue. Within the field of nursing, however, I have clues *if* I have knowledge and experience in that area with that type of an event.

Schools say they want to turn out critical thinkers, but they continue to use multiple guess questions to assess a student's knowledge and ability to reason. The average nurse has had 14 to 16 years of multiple guess questions throughout his schooling. He hits the patient care floor and we say, "*Now think!*" The student replies, "*What are my four options? One is really wrong, one is sorta wrong, one is really right, one is kinda right .....*" If this is how we train our students, how can we expect anything else?

In his book, *Developing Critical Thinkers*, Stephen Brookfield (1987) described the four components of critical thinking: 1) identifying and challenging assumptions; 2) challenging the importance of context; 3) imagining and exploring alternatives; and 4) reflective criticism. Critical thinking is also the ability to reason in a correct manner and to be able to identify false reasoning (McKinzie, 1992). These components elaborate on Watson and Glaser's definition of critical thinking and are integral parts of the whole process.

Facione (1990) defines critical thinking as: identifying and challenging assumptions, considering what is important in a situation, imaging and exploring alternatives, making informed decisions, and it is purposeful and goal oriented.

Identifying and Challenging Assumptions

We all make assumptions. A lot of us old nurses went to the class that taught us that to assume makes an "ass' out of "u" and "me." Consider the following scenario.

A man is standing outside his garage, watching it burn down. The fire department, paramedics, half the neighborhood, and this man's wife are all standing around watching the garage burn down. Suddenly the man clutches his chest and falls to the ground. What is wrong with him?

His heart? Do you know it is his heart? Is it an assumption on your part that it is his heart? An assumption, of course. Why did you need to make any assumption at all? Because it allows you to act. You must have a starting point. No assumption, no action.

Paramedics who witnessed the fall assumed the man was having a heart attack. They instituted ACLS and transported him the hospital. In the ER, the patient was very unstable. As was protocol, a nurse cut the patient's clothes off. The man was covered in hives.

Patients having MIs are not covered in hives. Patients having anaphylaxis to an allergen are covered in hives. The assumption that the man was having a heart attack allowed the paramedics to move into action. The new data that the man was covered in hives caused them to drop their first assumption, and move to the next assumption that it was anaphylaxis.

Assumptions allow you to act, but you have to know where you made them so you can make changes if new data proves them incorrect. A lot of us older nurses were taught that assumptions are bad and should not be made. If I ask an older nurse what assumptions were made in this situation, they frequently will reply strongly, "*None!*" Of course they made assumptions. If they didn't, there would be no action. Assumptions are not bad, because they allow you to act.

An assumption is your best guess based on your past experience as to what is happening. Your patient just threw up blood. What is your assumption? GI bleed? What in the world would make you think that someone who just threw up blood as having a GI bleed? Because every time you ever saw anyone throw up blood, it was due to a GI bleed. It is your best guess for a starting point. It is not necessarily the end, but rather a starting point for action. No assumption, no action.

Considering What is Important in a Situation

Salience is the ability to determine the important from the unimportant (Benner & Tanner, 1987). Novices have a very difficult time with this. To a novice, all data has the same importance; it is experience that teaches that some data is more important than others.

Imaging and Exploring Alternatives

There are so many different ways to get something done. There is no one, right way. Teachers need to open their students' minds to other possibilities. When someone is being taught a new skill, they need to be taught one way so they can learn, but after learning is achieved, there are many other possibilities. When initially learning Microsoft Word, the student doesn't want to hear that there are several options available for changing the font. They want to learn one way, when in fact there are several ways this task can be accomplished. The problem occurs if the teacher thinks that the way they are teaching is the "only way." The One and Only Way philosophy shuts down critical thinking in the student.

Making Informed Decisions

It is a sad fact that we know very little about how the human body works, what makes us sick, and what makes us well. We like to think we do, but in fact we know little. Nursing/medicine is a constantly shifting body of knowledge. What we "*know*" one year is wiped out by new research the next year. What this means is that we all must stay current on what the latest research shows and realize that new research tomorrow may obliterate today's knowledge. We are working with the best information we have at any given moment in time, but we need to be aware that, at any given moment in time, 50% of what we are doing is wrong. The problem is that we don't know which 50% it is! (It isn't called a practice for nothing.) You must stay current by going to lectures and presentations, reading journals, and talking with advanced practitioners.

Critical thinking is purposeful and goal oriented, but that does not mean it has to be difficult. If a patient is bleeding all over the floor, what is your goal for the patient? Stop the bleeding. The practitioner has to know where they are going, so they will know when they arrive. Also, if you don't have a goal, your therapy will be scattered and likely to be ineffective. There will be more on goals in the chapter on the Critical Thinking model.

Critical thinking may be many things to many people, but all will agree that it means making the *right* decision. In nursing, we are looking for the right decision in a clinical situation. We have already run into a problem. *Right* decision? Whose *right*? The doctor's right decision, the patient's son's right decision, the hospital administrator's right decision? No, the right decision for the patient. We want to do what minimizes harm and maximizes benefit to the patient. It sound easy, but can be very complex. In nursing, we want to stay within the current standards of established nursing practice while being our patient's advocate.

Requirements for Critical Thinking

Knowledge

The first requirement for critical thinking is knowledge. You cannot think about what you don't know. We all say we have a commitment to the education of our staff, but do we really? Does the nurse orienting the new person already have a full assignment of patients? Does just anyone who happens to be available that day do the orienting, or do you have a set program and competent, educated preceptors? Do staffing personnel routinely pull nurses out of educational offerings because they are easy to find there? Are nurses with educational days the first to be called back to work? Are educational events considered days off or days on the job? Is education a part of and an expectation of the job or a day off from real work? Florence Nightingale complained about her student nurses being pulled to the floor to work and never being able to properly complete their training. It is the same problem today. If you truly have a commitment to making your nurses into critical thinkers, the first item on the agenda is education.

I was contacted by a hospital to teach critical thinking to their nurses. I was to be allowed two hours to go over my model and the hospital decided to pass on the knowledge portion of the class. You cannot think critically about a subject when you lack knowledge. In this book, I have pulled together what I consider the essence of keeping a patient alive. If a nurse understands the effect of oxygen in the repolarization of the heart, s/he is more likely to remember to put oxygen on an unstable patient. If s/he understands that mottling of the skin is a sign of vasoconstriction seen with left heart failure, the doctor gets notified sooner. You only see what you know. You don't know it, there's no way you can see it. Nightingale said that if a nurse understands *why* she is doing something, she is more likely to be compliant with *what* the doctor wants done.

Experience

The second requirement for critical thinking to take place is experience. Experience is not time on the job, but rather how many times this event has happened to you in how many different subtle ways so that you can see it coming and know what to do about it. Experience is greatly augmented by mentoring. Novices need someone to help them understand situations. Assigning meaning is something parents do for their children; teachers do for their students. If someone is kind enough to tell you what that event means, you don't have to have it happen to you repeatedly before you finally figure out what the event means. All nurses should have someone they can turn to for explanations no matter how proficient they are.

The cogitative skills required for critical thinking are knowledge and experience. Knowledge is bits of data. When you come out of nursing school, your head is crammed full of bits of data. How many of you could pass the state boards tomorrow? None of us, but we are supposed to be superior to new grads who just passed state boards. What make us special? Pattern and context recognition. We see how things fit together and understand that things vary according to their context. We would never see patterns or understand context unless we first had the data (knowledge), but once we see patterns and context we can drop lots of the data. Which is why none of us could pass state boards at this point in our nursing careers but also why we function on a higher level than a new grad.

Knowledge without experience is dangerous. This is frequently the condition of a new grad. Experience without knowledge is equally as dangerous. Nurse's aides with years on the job can fit into this category. They know very well how to do a task, but have little to no understanding of why they are doing it or what it is meant to measure.

Environment

In order for critical thinking to take place, an environment needs to be present that supports it and a nurse who is inclined to do it. Critical thinking is a voluntary action. The person has to want to do it. But, assuming that a person is willing, it can only be done in a supportive environment. The thinker needs to have confidence that thinking independently will be fairly supported by nursing management. Thinking on your own is taking a risk. If the nurse feels that s/he will be hung out to dry should a conflict arise, they learn very quickly to stop thinking.

One concern that I hear over and over from preceptors is that the new orientee won't ask questions. If they don't ask questions, you can't ascertain their knowledge level. This is very frustrating for preceptors who need to know what the new nurse does or doesn't know so they can help fill in the blanks. If the new nurse won't ask questions, ask yourself if you have set up an environment where they feel safe asking questions. Not asking questions is a protective mechanism left over from nursing school. If the clinical instructor finds out that you don't know what you don't know, you can be asked to write a paper on it and present it to the class the next day, or possibly be ushered out the door. Nursing school is a very stressful situation that you are desperate to navigate, then pass your boards. At no time do you want to appear weak. Some of us take this so much to heart that we become incapable of asking questions.

Have you set up an environment that encourages questions? Is the new nurse fearful of losing her job if she isn't proficient, or does she feel you have a commitment to training and retaining her? Does she feel that she is out on a limb, or supported? Orienting to a new job is in some ways more stressful than nursing school and you need a certain degree of ego to ever think you could do something as complex and significant in other people's lives as being a nurse. That ego gets us up and off to the job every day, but it can also be a hindrance when we are the newbie and desperate to appear competent.

Observation from Inference

Critical thinkers need to be able to discriminate bias from reason and observation from inference. Did you actually see that happen or did you infer what happened based on your personal biases? We all have biases – they come from our past experience. Past experience is crucial to critical thinking, but past experience also places expectations on current events. We need to have a willingness to reconsider; this event may not be like the event that we experienced in the past. Always probe for assumptions based on past events.

Gaps in the Data

Be aware of gaps in the data. What is missing? What do I need before I act? If you have a patient with an arterial spurt, do you need more data before you act? An H&H? Set of vital signs? No more data is required! You need to put your finger on the dike. A patient complains of chest pain. Do you need more data before you mix the thrombolytic and inject it into the patient? Yes! Please don't do anything until you get more data. We have polar opposites here. One is act immediately and the other is please don't do anything until you get more data. These are extremes; most problems fall within the bell-shaped curve where you have some data and you are starting to act, but you are waiting for more data to come. Don't forget the missing data.

A patient is admitted to the CCU from the ER right at the change of shift – diagnosis: chest pain. All night long, the CCU nurses chased this lady's chest pain with nitrates, oxygen, morphine, and other therapies. They never made a dent in her chest pain unless she was snowed by the morphine.

About 6 a.m., the printer from the lab turned on and started printing out the day before's labs. At this point, the nurses realized that they had never seen this patient's admit labs. The patient had a hemoglobin of four, and that was the cause of her chest pain – myocardial ischemia secondary to severe anemia.

Don't forget the missing data; when it shows up it can change everything.

Always lobby for what is missing. Did we get the old chart yet? Has radiology read the X-ray? Are the labs back? How about the blood gas? He had a heart cath last week – where is the report? Missing data can hold the clue you've been looking for.

Masculine and Feminine Components

Critical thinking has components that are both masculine and feminine. Rationality is masculine. We love logic – because this is this and that is that, therefore this is that. Nice linear thinking; i.e., cause and effect. You can build decision trees based on this kind of information. We like it.

There are also feminine components to critical thinking – feelings, intuition and sensing. These come from our past experience. Nurses have always known that they had intuition, but they did not know how to explain it to anyone until two nurses, Benner and Tanner, did a study in 1987. They found that intuition was rapid critical thinking based on your past experience. Malcolm Gladwell based his 2005 book, *Blink: The Power of Thinking Without Thinking,* on these principals. Every time you had ever seen anyone look or act that way, nothing good ever came of it. So, intuition is based on past experience. This is why novices have no intuition – they have no past experience!

Pattern Recognition

Having the past experience isn't the whole entity; the nurse has to see and recognize patterns. This is why some people will never be good critical thinkers. You have to see patterns and recognize similarities between like events. An ability to see what is or is not important in a situation (salience) is crucial to critical thinking. Experienced nurses can do this very well, while novices do it poorly. Intuition mixes perception with proper action. You see it and do something about it.

Human beings sense and perceive much more that we think we do.

Just because we don't have a name for something doesn't mean it isn't there. The nurse who says, "*I just had a feeling so I acted*" is a wise nurse. Those feelings come from our past experience and should never be ignored. Intuition is your past experience talking to you – listen.

Components of Critical Thinking

- Specific knowledge base – for us it is nursing.
- Experience – nothing takes its place.
- Willingness – it is a voluntary action. You choose to think critically.
- Standards – because there are so many different ways to get something done.
- Somebody gets to say, "*No, that's wrong.*"

Our first set of standards comes from nursing school, your state boards or NCLEX exam. If you have professional certification, it comes with an expected standard of performance. Outside government agencies like JCAHO, HICFA, NOAH, or state inspectors are always happy to tell us what to do. There is quite a bit of leeway within the nursing standards of practice that allows for creativity to bring about a desired result, but there are definite standards of acceptability.

Critical thinking = knowledge + experience + willingness
Standards

Key Components to Chapter 14

1. Critical thinking requires knowledge, experience, a willingness to act, and a supportive environment.
2. Critical thinking requires guidelines for action. These are policies, procedures, guidelines and protocols.

Chapter 15

The Stages of Proficiency

In Benner's (1984/ 2001) landmark work, *From Novice to Expert*, she lists the stages a person goes through to become an expert at something. At first, we are novices at new tasks. About a year later, if we have had good experiences along with acquiring knowledge, we become advanced beginners. If things go well, a few years later we become competent in the job; later still, we may become proficient, and then, possibly, experts. No one is ever an expert at everything; we can be experts at something while only being advanced beginners in something else. Here, we will consider only the nursing profession, though any profession can be substituted; the first work with this model was actually done on airline pilots by Dreyfus and Dreyfus.

Stage 1: Novice

The first stage is that of novice – someone with little or no experience in this area. A novice's behavior is governed by rules, because he has little idea of what is relevant in a situation, and cannot grasp that meaning changes with context. Context, by itself, is a very hard concept to grasp and understanding only comes with wide experience. A novice doesn't have any experience, hence he also has no sense of context, no intuition, and no ability to be a critical thinker yet, as he has just begun his profession.

Experience is not merely the passage of time on the job. It implies that you have had many experiences with practical situations that add nuances or shades of differences, so that you can see a problem coming. Remember, you must do something seven times before you become accomplished. That's seven times for each and every skill you are trying to learn as a novice. Concepts and context come much further down the line.

Novices are rule-driven. They need things laid out clearly for them like a priority list: First do this, then do this, and then do that. This is because they are not capable of thinking outside of the box; they can't even see the box. But the problem with following rules is that rules can't tell the novice what is most important in any given situation. "...following rules legislates against successful performance because the rules cannot tell them the most relevant tasks to perform in an actual situation." (Benner, 2001, p. 21)

> I give instructions to the new graduate, very detailed and explicit instructions: When you come in first to see the baby, you take the baby's vital signs and make the physical examination, and you check the IV sites, and the ventilator and make sure it works, and you check the monitors and alarms. When I would say this to them, they would do exactly what I told them to do, no matter what else was going on .... They couldn't choose one thing to leave out. They couldn't choose what was the most important .... If I said you had to do these eight things ... they did those eight things. They couldn't choose what was most important. They didn't care if their other kid was screaming his head off. When they did realize, they would be like a mule between two piles of hay (Benner, 2001).

Novices are rule-driven, so we must teach them this way. They cannot move on to the stages of proficiency until they have the rules down pat. Everything will be built on a foundation of knowledge. Only after the knowledge is acquired can the nurse move up the stages of proficiency. Novices do not understand concepts, only facts. Concepts come later.

Data missed in orientation can cause problems later on. Because you don't want to leave anything out, formal precepting programs are the most efficient way of making sure knowledge is distributed. If you leave the teaching up to a scattering of teachers without formal guidelines of content, I can guarantee that holes will be discovered in the novice nurse's learning at the least opportune time. ("But, no one ever *told* me that!" is heard way too often.)

When instructors make up class content, remember to prioritize what your novice needs to know in order to function efficiently, on the night shift, with Dr. Obnoxious ranting in the background.

Stage 2: Advanced Beginner

After about a year, the nurse shows marginally acceptable performance and has coped with enough real situations to begin seeing the importance of context. Context can only be seen through the lens of prior experience. When there was no prior experience, there cannot be a comparison of how a given patient is similar to – or different than – others. Benner uses the example of an advanced beginner nurse accessing a patient's readiness to learn about his new ostomy:

> Earlier I thought he was feeling hopeless about the operation he had just had. He looked as though he felt crummy – physically, sort of stressed looking, nervous looking. Furthermore he was treating the wound very gingerly. He didn't need to be that gentle with it. But on this morning, it was different; he began to ask questions about his care. (p. 22)

A novice would have begun teaching immediately because it was time to teach, or it was a task that needed to be done. The advanced beginner nurse knows patients don't learn until they are ready to learn and looks for signs of readiness before beginning to impart knowledge. Context has become important.

Because the advanced beginner sees context, they should now be able to follow clinical guidelines. These guidelines require the nurse to understand that all patients and situations are not the same. Guidelines are guides – they do not by any means cover all clinical situations. The nurse has to know what principles the guidelines are talking about look and sound like when dealing with real people. Experience is what helps a nurse learn, while mentoring greatly enhances the value of experience. The main difference between a novice and an advanced beginner is that a novice cannot follow guidelines because they are too busy trying to remember the rules they have just learned.

Advanced beginners still need a great deal of help in clinical settings with setting priorities and seeing patterns. They are much more accomplished than novices, but still cannot prioritize conflicting tasks, and they don't understand the importance, or lack thereof (salience), of all of the data swirling around them. Because of this, advanced beginner nurses still need the guidance of a nurse more advanced in nursing practice.

Stage 3: Competent

After two to three years of experience, nurses may become competent. The competent nurse is skilled with tasks, understands context, and is able to set long range goals for the patient. What most characterizes this level of proficiency is a written plan for the day's activities; conscious, deliberate planning and an increase in efficiency characterize the competent nurse.

Benner uses the following example of a nurse going from advanced beginner to competent:

I had four patients. One needed colostomy teaching; the others needed a lot of other things. When I went out there, instead of thinking when I went into the room ... you get caught up ... someone's IV stops, and you get caught up working on that. And then you forget to give someone their meds, and you have to rush around and do that. And then someone is feeling nauseated and you try to make them feel better while they are sick. And then the colostomy bag falls off and you want to start teaching them. All of a sudden the morning is gone and no one has gotten a bed bath.

Now I come out of report and know what their IVs are basically, and I have a couple of things that I know I have to do. Before I go into the room I write down what meds I'm supposed to give for that day, and then I'll walk in there and make sure everyone's IVs are fine. You go from bed to bed and say just say "Hi" and introduce yourself. But I give them the message that I am attending to business. I check their IVs, check their dressings. And then I feel fine. I know they are not going to bleed to death; I know the urine output is OK; I know that their IVs are fine … then I have the whole morning set out and I can go ahead and do things. I am much more organized. I know what I have to do, and I arrange it with them and find out what they want to do. (p. 26)

The competent nurse lacks the speed and flexibility of a nurse in the higher stages of proficiency, but the clinical world has become organized after great effort on their part. A conscious, deliberate plan helps to achieve that efficiency and organization.

Stage 4: Proficient

The proficient nurse sees the whole picture, not merely a set of tasks to be accomplished. Things must be done, sure, but they are done to enhance the patient's movement from point A to point B. The proficient nurse is able to match patterns. They think, "Is this patient acting as they should in this circumstance? Have other patients been like this or different from this patient when in the same situation?" Perspective is not thought out, but rather "presents itself" based on experience and recent events. The proficient nurse learns to expect what might go wrong, then acts accordingly. He is able to recognize the nuances of a situation because he has had a great deal of experience. It takes at least three to five years to reach this stage (if the nurse ever does). It takes *time*.

The proficient nurse is the bane of the nurse educator. At this stage of practice, nursing theory becomes useless – mere trappings. This type of nurse views the nurse educator's elaborate decision analysis as an unnecessarily excessive way to solve a clinical problem the nurse can now grasp quickly.

When the learner advances to concepts, he tends to forget how complex the learning process was to get to those concepts.

When the light goes on and he suddenly "sees" the answer, he thinks this was all he needed to know in the first place, when, in fact, "seeing" was the end of a long learning process that began at the novice stage. This is why proficient nurses want to describe complex subtleties to the novice, who has no idea what they are talking about. This is the nurse who may pull a novice to the side and say, "You don't need to know that. This is what you *really* need to know." These nurses think they are making things easier and simpler for the novice, not realizing that the rules and decision making models are the basis for later understanding.

Only by dropping the rules can one become truly proficient, but you must *know* the rules to *become* proficient. Deviating from the rules can increase productivity, but a firm grasp of the rules and an understanding of nuance is necessary. Benner has an example of the complexities of the clinical situation and how the proficient nurse thinks:

> Well, you look at their vital signs to see if anything is significant ... but even then you need to do a little guessing, in terms of whether the patient is just anxious because he is so used to the machine breathing for him ... If they get a little anxious, you don't really want to medicate them because you are afraid they might quit breathing, but on the other hand they may really need to calm down a little bit, so it just depends on the situation. It is a real experiment. You have your groundwork from what you have done in the past, and you know when you are going to get into trouble. (p. 29)

The proficient nurse understands salience and sees when the expected norm is not materializing quickly enough. Because of his vast experience, he doesn't so much "plan" as just know what to do; it becomes an unconscious, rather than conscious, effort. These nurses run on maxims that are context-driven. Nuance is everything to the proficient nurse.

Stage 5: Expert

The expert nurse does not use rules, guidelines, or maxims, but rather operates from a deep understanding of the situation, based on years and years of practical experience. Expert nurses exhibit an intuitive grasp of the clinical situation, zeroing right in on the problem. They operate from deep understanding of the total situation ("it felt right," or "it looked good"). Dreyfus and Dreyfus (1977) explain it this way: The performer is no longer aware of the features and rules of his/her performance and the performance becomes fluid and flexible and highly proficient. The chess player develops a feel for the game; the language learner becomes fluent; the pilot stops feeling that he/she is flying the plane and simply feels he/she is flying. (p. 12). Here is an expert nurse responding to a bleeding patient in Benner:

I had worked late and was just about ready to go home, when a nurse preceptor said to me, "Jolene, come here." Her voice had urgency in it, but not Code Blue. I walked in and I looked at the patient and his heart rate was about 120, and he was on the respirator and breathing. And I asked her: "What's wrong?" There was a new graduate taking care of him. And he just pointed down to the patient who was lying in a pool of blood. There was a big stream of blood drooling out of his mouth. This man's diagnosis was mandibular cancer which had been resected, and about a week previous to that, he had had a carotid bleed from the external carotid which had been ligated secondary to radiation erosion. That wound had become septic and he had developed respiratory failure and he was in ICU for that. So I looked at the dressing and it was dry, the blood was coming out of his mouth. The man had a tracheotomy because of the type of surgery that had been done. He also had an NG tube in for feedings, and I got to thinking that it might be the innominate or the carotid artery that had eroded. So we took him off the ventilator to see if anything was going to pump out of the trach. There was a little blood, but it looked mostly like it had come down from the pharynx into the lungs. So we began hand ventilating him, trying to figure out what the devil was inside his mouth that was pumping out this tremendous amount of blood.

By this time the problem is blood, we need blood, and so I said, "OK, someone call the blood bank and get some blood." And the nurse said, "We just called and there's none down there." No one had caught that the patient was sitting up there with no blood in the blood bank. So we took off a blood from the arterial line and sent it down for a type and cross match.

Meanwhile, I started Plasmanate and lactated Ringers, because the mean pressure was dropping down to about 30 and the blood was just pumping out of his mouth. About this time the ICU resident came in and looked bewildered like "what are we going to do?" He asked if we had an ancillary line in. I said, "Yes, we have a central venous pressure line in, but I don't think that's going to be enough." He said "I'll do a cutdown." I said, "I don't think you have to; I think I can get one in." So I took a 14-gauge and put it into the intracubital space. There are two plasmas going in. He said, "What shall I do?" And I said, "You need to go down to the blood bank and get some type-specific blood for this patient, because a nurse can't get that. You are the only person who can get type-specific blood." I said, "Bring two units; they will only give you two at a time, no matter how bad. But bring two and get back here as soon as you can." So he took off.

This is a novice nurse's view of the same event.

This man is a very pleasant fellow, very bright, very alert and awake, and was unfortunately requiring tracheal suctioning approximately every hour to two hours for moderate amounts of tracheal secretions which were relatively tenacious in character, relatively white tannish in color. He unfortunately did not tolerate the suctioning extremely well. It was relatively uncomfortable for him, caused a moderate amount of cough and gag reflex, which in turn caused a transient increase in blood pressure. Following suctioning on one occasion, as I was replacing his tracheal mist mask he began coughing copious amounts of bright red blood per mouth. I mildly panicked, called for help from the nurse next door, placed him in a moderate Trendelenberg position, opened his IV to a rapid rate, and continued to experience mild panic. Perhaps more like moderate panic.

The difference between these two nurses' reactions is like night and day. But, remember that it is knowledge, experience, and a desire to advance that makes an expert. We want our novices to come out of orientation as proficient, or even better, expert nurses, but it isn't possible. Proficiency takes time and hands-on experience.

An interesting thing about experts is that if they are faced with a situation where they have no previous experience or things are not turning out like expected, they revert promptly to the analytical skills used at the lower levels of proficiency. Move any experienced nurse into a new or different area of practice and they will become novices again. Because of his vast knowledge, however, he will move through the stages of proficiency much faster than someone just entering nursing. First it is rules, then concepts, followed by seeing, and finally, knowing.

All nurses are not the same; they are at different levels of proficiency. The different stages require different teaching strategies to help nurses grow.

All classification systems are oversimplifications that barely reflect reality. We have the components of several different learning styles and are never all at any one stage, but rather an expert at this and a novice at that. These classifications are useful to help us so we can understand how to teach nurses at every level and stage to become more effective.

Key Components in Chapter 15

1. There are levels of proficiency that we all go through when we orient to a new job or environment.
2. We must teach learners based on their level of proficiency.
3. Experience is not years on the job; it is how many times you have had this experience in how many different ways so that you can see it coming.

Chapter 16

A Critical Thinking Model

Whenever a person problem-solves, they should have a set way of attacking the problem. Problem-solving is a mental discipline that allows for analyzing all the facts before making a decision. If I am teaching students to interpret EKG rhythms, they are told they will analyze each strip in exactly the same way. Are there p waves? How many ps per QRS? What is the pr interval? And so on, until every facet of the heart rhythm is looked at before making a decision. Otherwise, they might just look at the strip and say, *"Oh, that's a Mobitz II"* and be wrong at the least opportune time. This mental discipline needs to be carried over to critical thinking. There needs to be a set way of looking at a problem so that no facts are left out or overlooked before a decision is made. The next part of this book looks at a model that promotes critical thinking in the clinical setting.

A novice and experienced nurse are caring for a patient at the bedside when something goes wrong. The experienced nurse steps in and fixes the problem. After the event is over the novice says to the experienced nurse, *"Why did you do that therapy?"* and the experienced nurses says, *"That's what you are supposed to do."* This makes the novice crazy. She cannot go from event to therapy and she feels she is so dumb that she will never learn how to be good nurse. Her anxiety level goes up, her learning goes down, and the experienced nurse says, *"She just doesn't get it."*

When Benner, et. al., studied the stages of proficiency, they realized that at the higher proficiencies, nurses were like onions. There were many layers that needed to be peeled away in order to see the thought process that went into decision-making. The experienced nurse didn't really say, *"That's what you are supposed to do."* They had actually looked carefully at the problem, different things that could be causing the problem, different things they could do about the problem, what would be the good or the bad of each choice, chosen something, acted on it, and weren't even aware that they had done all of this before reaching a decision. In order for the novice to learn from a more experienced nurse, the first thing you have to do is you must slow the experienced nurse's thought process down to where the novice can see it. The following model for critical thinking does just that.

Whiteside's Critical Thinking Model

- Problem:
  - » current:
  - » potential:
- Data:
- Assumptions:
- Reasons:
- Goals:
- Methods:
- + and – side effects of each:

Problem

If you are going to problem-solve, the first step is to determine what the **problem** is. Experienced nurses do this very well; novices do it very poorly. Again, it is an experience thing. Problems come in two kinds: **current** and **potential**. A current problem is something that is *happening right now* that is a problem for this patient. These include abnormal vital signs, organ dysfunction, co-morbid factors, drugs in the patient that should or should not be there, bleeding, etc.

Potential problems are ones that will occur in the future if something isn't done to change the current situation. The experienced nurse looks immediately into the future and says, "*Oh, no!*" and does something to fix the current problem so the potential problem never occurs. The novice nurse doesn't know how to look into the future and is unaware of any potential problem until it happens. This part of the model teaches the novice to look into the future for potential complications.

Missing Data

The next component to the model looks at **missing data**. What would you like to know about this situation? *"Where is the doctor?"* is not an option at this stage unless the nurse is a novice. Some nurses cannot think past, *"Call the doctor!"* I like to ask experienced nurses if they've figured out what their job as a nurse is yet. Most aren't too sure because the job is so diverse. I see the nurse as the Great Suggester. It is the nurse who says to the doctor, *"Have you considered, would you like, how about?"* You can't have any idea what to suggest unless you know what you should be suggesting. Beyond the novice level, nurses need to have a good idea of what the doctors need to be ordering. In fact, nurses have been held legally responsible for knowing if the doctor wrote the right order.

In the missing data section is everything you would like to know about the situation. Pertinent information – things like vital signs trends, physical exam, lab tests, H&P, results of procedures and tests recently completed and not on the chart yet, X-rays, EKGs, ABGs, family input, the patient's description of the problem, what makes it better, what makes it worse, etc. Data you need in order to form an opinion on what might be going on. Ranking is of importance in the data section of the model; how do you know what to do first? There are so many possibilities. You do not want to tell the novice to do this, then this, then this. That stops all critical thinking. Novices and advanced beginners are so rule-driven that they will not be able to see past the directions if there is a variance from the norm.

Critical thinking is about possibilities, so you want as many possibilities to come into the picture as possible, but some are more important than others and should be done first. The data to be obtained includes: ct scan of chest, physical exam, patient's list of medications, blood work, old chart, vital signs, SPO2, blood cultures, H&P, ER record, urinalysis, and EKG. What is the first to be done? All are important, but how do they rank in order of consequence?

We must prove that the patient is oxygenating and perfusing at the same time. For oxygenation, I have O2 sat, vital signs, and physical exam. Those things tell you if the patient is oxygenating. For perfusion, there is the EKG, vital signs, and physical exam. The most important things to get done are the physical exam, EKG, O2 sat, and vital signs. This is exactly what you do for these patients every day. Rather than telling the student what to do, we have let them come to their own conclusion and have not shut down thinking about other possibilities. They now have an order for their actions that makes sense to them.

Assumptions

Next, what **assumptions** have you made? You must make an assumption as a starting point for action. Our assumption might not turn out to be true, but it is a starting point. It is your first blush guess as to what is going on. The patient just vomited bright red blood. What is your assumption? Based on your past experience, what is your best guess? A GI bleed? A good starting assumption. It may turn out to be a nose bleed and the patient swallowed the blood, but a GI bleed is a logical starting point.

What else could be causing this problem? What other **reasons** could there be for this to be happening? Every event has multiple things that could be causing it to happen. You have a patient with no heart rate. How many things can you think of that would cause a patient to not have a heart rate? To your list, add being frozen in a block of ice, or a gunshot wound to the left ventricle. Were those on your list? How about a disconnected EKG lead? There are multiple things that could be causing anything to occur. This part of the model is called hypothesis generation, otherwise known as possibilities. The more hypotheses that are generated, the more likely the right one will arrive. Experienced nurses do it very well; novices do it poorly. Because you cannot think of what you do not know, it is experience that drives this section.

Goal of Therapy

What is the patient care **goal**? What are you trying to accomplish? Students need to know what it is they are trying to accomplish. Is it to get the blood pressure up, or stop the bleeding, or get a new drug ordered? You have to know what it is you are trying to do so you can know if you are headed in the right direction. Otherwise, your therapy is scattered rather than concentrated in one or two directions. Understanding this section of the model is crucial for moving on to the methods section.

Our goal for patient care is always that the patient be oxygenating and perfusing at the same time. To determine the goal, look in the current problem list and see what is keeping the patient from oxygenating and perfusing at the same time. Let's say the blood pressure is down. Will that keep the patient from oxygenating and perfusing at the same time? Yes. What is your goal? To get the blood pressure back up. We are now all on the same page and can move forward together.

Remember that you are talking to novices. Do not use big, flowery terms when you are talking to novices. Big, flowery terms impede learning. If you tell me "*tachepnea,*" I think "*tachepnea, tachepenea ... now which one is that? Is it the calcium or the potassium?*" Your explanation is way down the line as I am stuck on "*What is tachepnea?*" Use words like heart rate up or blood pressure down – things everyone understands. You are supposed to be trying to teach me, not impress me.

Methods for Achieving the Goal

The final section is **methods**. How are you going to go about achieving your goal? This section is, as are all the others, about possibilities. What are the possible options for action? You should never do anything to anyone unless you know what could result from your action – the good and the bad. Let's say the patient's blood pressure is down and your goal is to get the blood pressure back up. One method that could be used is a bolus of IV fluid. The good thing that could happen is that the patient's blood pressure goes up. The bad things are fluid overload, congestive heart failure, pulmonary edema, and death from a lethal dysrythmia. For every method there are positive and negative consequences, what I call the positive and negative spillover effects.

The method section is all of the possible things you can think of to meet the goal. This section is answered based on the nurse's skill level and job experience. If a patient's father is having a heart attack in OB, the proper answer for the OB nurse will include administering O2 and calling for help. But if the heart attack occurs in the CCU, the proper response would include the ACLS algorithm for AMI.

When all the possible methods and their good and bad side effects are listed, you ask the student to choose which one to do first and justify his answer. This is what the experienced nurse did in his head, totally unaware that he had gone through this entire process. Have the novice explain why he would or would not use each of the methods and justify his decision.

When there are multiple possibilities or variables, how do you know what is the most important or which one to go for first? Which of the possibilities should be the assumption? The first one to eliminate is the one that will kill the patient, then the one that will maim the patient. Everything else comes after those two have been eliminated. Things that keep the patient from oxygenating and perfusing at the same time should be eliminated first. For a patient with crushing chest pain, possibilities could be ACS or a gall bladder attack. It is the myocardial infarction that will kill the patient first. Eliminate the heart and you have the rest of the patient's life to look at his gut. Eliminate the gut first and you may have a dead patient.

Key Components to Chapter 16

1. Novices' critical thinking abilities will increase if you give them a framework within which to work.
2. When making a decision, one needs to consider what the problem is, what data is missing, what assumptions have been made, what else could be causing this to happen, what is the goal of therapy, and any and all methods for achieving the goal, complete with the positive and negative spillover effects of each method.
3. Novices' critical thinking abilities increase if you give them a framework within which to work.

Effectiveness of the Model

The effectiveness of the model was evaluated with a small sample of students in a pre-experimental study (Table 1). The study utilizing the model for teaching critical thinking explored whether these skills could be changed in as little as 10 weeks. Students' critical thinking abilities were measured with the Watson – Glazer Critical Thinking Appraisal (WGCTA) before and after taking a 10 week critical care course (Table 2). The course was given to experienced, working nurses who wished to improve their clinical skills. The course presented a knowledge base and utilized the model/scenario/debate approach to teaching critical thinking.

The results (Table 3) showed a significant improvement in the critical thinking scores of the test group (paired t -3.33, df 26, p .003). It was the students who initially showed the least ability to think critically (the lower third of the WGCTA scores) who showed a vast improvement in their scores.

Limitations of the Study

This study was limited due to its small sample group. The study should be repeated with a larger sample and more diverse groups.

Results

The results of the study suggest that critical thinking skills can be improved by using the model. The fact that improvement was seen in scores with only a 10-week time period implies that this model can be applied to all types of nursing – whether it is a program lasting one hour or several years. Students received immediate feedback with regard to their choices and the scenario's outcome. This is a format that lends itself easily to computer assisted learning and allows critical thinking skills to be incorporated into any and all form of nursing education.

Example

A novice nurse performed less that ideally when her patient went into respiratory distress. She focused on one symptom (as novices are known to do) and did not see all that was going on with the patient. In this instance, it was a lack of knowledge, as well as a lack of critical thinking. Remember, you can't think critically if you don't have the data. . The preceptor turned the situation into a learning experience. The model became a lesson plan for teaching and a framework for discussion to take place. The preceptor was able to ascertain what knowledge the novice lacked, teach it, and discuss the patient situation in a constructive, non-threatening way.

Design

The study used a pre-experimental design because there was no control group. The assumption was that the control group would not have changed their critical thinking scores without the teaching. The study group was given the WGCTA pre- and post- the 10-week class. Two different WGCTAs were used to eliminate an improvement in scores based on an acquired familiarity with the testing method.

Sample

The sample for the study was a convenience sample comprised of students in a critical care course who agreed to participate. Thirty-five nurses began the course; twenty-seven nurses comprised the study group at the end of the course. The sample was varied in terms of age, years of nursing experience, entry level into nursing, and specialty certification (Table 2).

Instrumentation

Critical thinking was evaluated using the WGCTA, as it is designed to measure generic critical thinking ability and does not require knowledge in any one particular content area. The instrument tests an individual's ability to define a problem, select pertinent information, recognize stated and unstated assumptions, formulate a relevant hypothesis, draw valid conclusions, and judge the validity of inferences. Form A of the WGCTA was used as the pre-course assessment tool and Form B was used as the post-course tool.

A pre- and post-course knowledge exam was used to test the students' general acquisition. The pre-test determined how much knowledge the students had of the course material before the class began (Table 1). Knowledge and critical thinking scores were then compared (Table 3).

Data Collection

The initial administration of the WGCTA and the knowledge test took place at the beginning of the first day of class. At this time, a demographic questionnaire was also filled out by the students (Table 2). The class was then taught over 10 weeks and used the model/scenario/debate technique for imparting critical thinking skills along with the normal class content. On the last day of the class, the WGCTA and the same knowledge test was re-administered to the students.

Data Analysis

Differences in the pre- and post-class WGCTA scores were examined by a paired t test. WGCTA post-course scores were significantly higher than pre-course scores (t = -3.33, df = 26, p = .003). Change in the knowledge test scores were also looked at using the paired t test and reflected the knowledge the student had learned in the class (t = -9.96, df = 26, p = .000). Table 1 summarizes the WGCTA and knowledge test scores.

Finally, the relationship between the student's pre- and post-course WGCTA and pre- and post-course knowledge scores was explored. A Person's r was performed and only a weak and statically non-significant (r = .18) correlation was found. Analysis showed that subjects with lower scores on the pre-course WGCTA tended to show more extreme positive changes in their post-course scores ($r = -.68$, $p < .01$). The students most in need of improvement in their critical thinking skills gained the most from the use of the model.

Discussion of Findings

Results for the study suggest that critical thinking skills can be improved. Statistically significant changes occurred in knowledge acquisition and critical thinking skills in the study group. The nurses with the highest pre-course WGCTA scores showed the least improvement in their critical thinking skills. This suggests that these techniques are the most helpful in those nurses who need it most. It is in this group of students that nurse educators would like to see the most improvement.

Table 1. WGCTA and Knowledge Scores Pre and Post-course					
WGCTA			Knowledge		
pre	post	change	pre	post	change
71	70	-1	76	88	+12
55	66	+11	55	84	+29
57	56	-1	55	84	+29
67	71	+4	57	78	+21
42	47	+7	55	84	+29
40	46	+6	27	85	+58
46	56	+10	42	90	+48
58	57	-1	45	75	+10
53	45	-8	57	67	+10
61	59	-2	60	70	+10
40	49	+10	37	55	+18
50	55	+5	67	93	+26
27	54	+27	79	87	+8
38	60	+22	51	85	+34
67	61	-6	48	84	+36
59	58	-1	67	88	+21
57	64	+7	40	73	+33
58	57	-1	66	79	+13
59	59	0	58	91	+33
51	73	+22	45	82	+37
39	52	+13	70	76	+6
40	52	+12	34	75	+41
35	60	+25	40	85	+45
56	47	-9	43	84	+11
58	61	+3	64	88	+24
67	69	+2	61	76	+15
42	60	+18	67	73	+6
MEANS					
51.6	57.9	+5.22	54.0	80.7	+26.4

Table 2. Characteristics of the Sample		
Characteristic	Sample size	% of sample
Gender		
male	1	3.7
female	26	96.3
Nursing degree		
Diploma	3	11.1
ADN	17	63.0
BSN	7	25.9
Certification		
Yes	7	25.9
No	20	74.1
Previous logic class		
Yes	4	14.8
No	23	85.2
Previous CCU course		
Yes	5	18.5
No	22	81.5
Age		
Mean = 40.5 (+/- 9.8)		
Range = 22 to 55		
Years of nursing experience		
Mean = 9.5 (+/- 7.21)		
Range = 0 to 22		

Table 3. Changes in Pre and Post-Course WGCTA and Knowledge Test Scores				
t – test for Paired Samples				
Test	Pre-course mean	Post-course mean	t (df = 26)	p
WGCTA	51.6 +/- 11.35	57.9 +/- 7.68	-3.33	.003
Knowledge	54.3 +/- 13.2	80.7 +/- 8.4	-9.96	.000

Key Components in Chapter 17

1. The model is effective in teaching critical thinking skills, especially to the students who possessed the lowest critical thinking abilities in the beginning.
2. It has to be used consistently in order to work.

Chapter 18
Teaching Critical Thinking

Experience shows us patterns, how things are linked together, and that some things are more important than others. Junior nursing students will rank constipation and 3rd degree heart block with the same importance in their drug cards. Though both are complications of beta blockers, the 3rd degree heart block is of course more important. The nursing student understands constipation, but may not yet grasp the intricacies of heart blocks.

We are always trying to make sense of our world and to put it into shapes and forms we understand. This is why adult learners learn best when new information is added to already existing knowledge. This is also why the best teaching makes use of the student's current understanding of how the world works. Everyone understands how a toilet flushes and that if you don't allow the tank to fill, the next flush will only have a partial volume and strength. If the teacher equates that to the filling and emptying of the heart, then the student easily understands that premature beats have less volume and pressure, and that less pulse can be felt at the wrist.

When teaching critical thinking, it is important for the teacher and student to understand that critical thinking is about possibilities. What courses of action are possible in a given situation? Not "*what do I do,*" but "*what are the possibilities?*" If one teaches a person to do step one, then step two, then step three, all critical thinking is lost. As previously stated, novices are incredibly rule-driven. If a teacher says one, two, three, novices are not capable of looking beyond that when the situation changes. They simply do not know what to do.

I went to a code one day and I was the first person in the room. I looked around and there was no one in the room but me and the dead lady lying on the bed. I was very puzzled as I thought we were having a code in this room. Pretty soon, here came both novice nurses pushing the code cart. They knew that the first thing you did in a code was to put oxygen on the patient. They looked and they didn't have a flow meter. Because number one on the list of things to do in a code was oxygen, they did not know what else to do. So, both of them left the patient and went down the hall to get the code cart. There was a flow meter on the code cart (it took both of them in case the cart tipped over) and back they came. By this time, the entire code team was standing in the patient's room wondering if there was really a code or not.

This is the kind of behavior you get when you teach one, two, and three. We teach A, B, C: airway, breathing, and circulation for codes. That is fine, but novices and advanced beginners don't have the experience to see past that. If you have everything you need, great. But what if something is missing? An experienced nurse would never have left the code patient's bedside if there was no flow meter. S/he would have tried another tactic; if it didn't work, then s/he would have tried something else, but the experienced nurse would *never* have left the patient.

So, don't teach one, two, and three. Teach instead *"here is our goal, and here are our possibilities. What you do depends on what you have available and what is appropriate in this patient care situation."* This keeps the door open for critical thinking. Algorithms slam the door on thinking, which is why there are very few of them in the new ACLS books. Instead of *"do this, do this, and do this,"* they say, *"have you considered, maybe try this, or here is a possibility."* We like to be told what to do in a crisis, but in fact we are all different and no two events are exactly alike. It requires critical thinking to see the variables and patterns.

Nothing in nursing/medicine is linear. It always depends on co-morbid factors, complications, what drugs are on board (or should be on board, but are not), the status of the patient's kidneys and liver today, how much stress has he been under, what the patient's reserves are, etc. It depends on everything and no algorithm can take all of that into account. Only the human brain can, with knowledge and experience.

Teaching "do this, do this, do that" slams the door on critical thinking. There must be guidelines for treatment, but there must also be opportunity for variances from the norm.

Key Components in Chapter 18
1. Critical thinking is about possibilities.
2. Don't teach: do 1, do 2, do 3. It slams the door on critical thinking.
3. Teach: here is our goal of therapy and here are possibilities.
4. What you do depends on what you have available and what is applicable to this patient in this context.

Chapter 19

Examples Using the Critical Thinking Model

Garbage Pile

You have just moved into a real fixer-upper home. It has possibilities, but it needs a lot of work. Numerous things need to be done to the house, but the yard has its own problems – it has been used as a dumping ground for debris from home building and repair and toxic waste of paints and cleaning chemicals, as well as car parts and tree stumps.

Problems:

Current – stuff is where you don't necessarily want it: toxic chemicals

Potential – injury, fines, complaints from neighbors, disease, rodents

What More Data is Necessary?

What are the contents of the debris and waste; where can it be taken and how much will it cost; cost of someone doing it for you; what is recyclable and/or valuable; who is responsible to pay for and make the cleanup; what are the rules for disposal of these types of things; do you have a truck; do you know someone with a big enough truck; does anyone owe you a favor; are your sons home; etc.

Assumption

It is bad and needs to be fixed.

Other Possible Reasons for the Problem

Poor planning and completion on the part of the last homeowner; it is the neighborhood's custom; it isn't debris, but rather home improvement supplies; it is a good thing and a sign of status to have this in your yard; a tornado hit your yard.

Goal
Clean up the mess.

Methods
1. Do it yourself.
   The good thing here is that it can be done on your time schedule, done to your specifications, and might cost less. The downside is that it is your time, your money, your muscle, and your exposure; you may do it wrong or hurt yourself.
2. Have someone else do it.
   This one gets it done, but it is expensive and may not be precisely what you wanted done or get accomplished on your time schedule.
3. Bury it.
   Again, it's gone, but this may not be legal, toxic chemicals can leech into the groundwater, and you can find yourself with a fine or worse.
4. Burn it where it lays.
   It is gone, but done illegally. The burning can harm other people, causing you to receive a fine from the fire department, and it might burn your house down if you include a little bad luck into the mix.
5. Force the previous home owner to make it right.
   It is gone; the legal action may cost you money, cause aggravation, and stress.
6. Cover it with dirt, plant grass, put in a skateboard park on the steep parts, and charge admission.
   Now it is no longer a problem and you can make money off the deal, but it is illegal; you have only covered over the problem, can be fined, and you will damage the environment.

I particularly liked the last answer, "make a skateboard park," as a method. That the debris could actually be home improvement supplies was suggested by various students. These ideas are not ridiculous, but rather show creativity on the part of the learner.

Critical thinking requires that all possibilities be considered. When circumstances change, the ridiculous can become just the right thing to do. When the teacher shuts down creativity, they have shut off thinking. These are the kinds of thinking proficient and expert nurses can do, but we must begin teaching it to the novice so it can survive into later stages of proficiency. Close the door to creativity now and it may never reappear again.

When answering a patient care scenario, it is important to remember that the student should answer from the perspective of his proficiency level and work area. Those in differing levels of proficiency answer with differing degrees of expertise, and OB nurses have a different frame of reference from that of CCU nurses. Context is everything. A drop in hematocrit in an ante- to post-partum mom is different from a drop of the hematocrit in an Acute Coronary Syndrome patient post-thrombolytic therapy.

Jack

Jack is a 65-year-old man presenting in the ER after crushing chest pain awoke him at 2 a.m. When the paramedics arrived, they were able to relieve the pain with nitrates and oxygen. In the ER, his vital signs were B/P 120/60, HR 88, RR 16, he was in sinus rhythm, and has an IV of D5W at a TKO rate of 50 cc per hour. A cardiologist sees Jack and begins him on Lopressor10 mg po q 6 hours. He is transferred to your work area. (Wherever you work, Jack is in your work area.) Answer the questions from the standpoint of your work area.

At 11 a.m., Jack calls you and complains of 5/10 chest pain and "not feeling well." His B/P is 104/50 and his HR is 65. You give him 1 tab of NTG sublingual and within one minute his vital signs plunge to: B/P 70/40, HR 42, RR 34, and he is pale, cold, clammy, and diaphoretic.

Problem: Current

The heart rate and blood pressure are down, the respiratory rate is up, the patient is cold, clammy, and diaphoretic. These are the easily defined problems. There are in fact three other major problems for Jack that are so blatant and so obvious that the experienced nurse immediately adds them into their thought process without being aware they have done so – and the novice can't see it happen. It is important that all the problems be expressed. The patient's subjective feeling is here – "I don't feel well." This is vital information. Teach your novice to listen to the patient. If the patient says it isn't right, it isn't right. If the patient's family says it isn't right, it isn't right.

Two other problems are the patient's admission diagnosis of recent chest pain and the fact that he has Lopressor and NTG in his body. Any drug a patient has in his body is a problem. Any drug he should have in his body that he doesn't have in his body is a problem. Lopressor is particularly nasty as it is a beta blocker and will mask the physiological signs of compensation in the patient's body.

Problems: Potential

What will happen to Jack if we don't do anything about the current problems? A lethal dysrhythmia and death. I have found that novices will do better if you step them through a process rather than asking for a leap of faith. So how do you go from low heart rate and blood pressure to dead? It's very fast, but there are steps in the process. The decreased heart rate and BP cause a decrease in perfusion into the tissues. The decreased perfusion decreases the amount of oxygen being delivered. The cells go anaerobic, stop functioning as they should, and start cranking out lactic acid. Lactic acid causes a lactic acidosis and changes the body's pH. The four things that can cause a lethal dysrythmia are: 1. Change in pH, 2. Imbalance in electrolytes, 3. Hypoxia, and 4. Insufficient glucose in the cell to make ATP. Also, the lesser amount of blood and oxygen into the heart does not allow the action potential to be successful, the heart is not repolarized after being depolarized, and a lethal dysrythmia ensues.

What More Data is Needed?

Everything you would like to know about the situation. We will focus the student into the most important things after we have brainstormed about possibilities. Remember, critical thinking is about possibilities, not do this, this, and this. I would like an EKG, the old chart and an old EKG to compare to the current one, H&P, medication list with allergies, more info about the chest pain (what makes it better, what makes it worse), CXR, I&O + weight, BUN Cr, CBC, O2 sat, ABG, head-to-toe physical exam, vital signs, heart enzymes, BNP, lytes, toxicology screen, H&P, code status, heart echo, d-dimer, ct spiral, etc.

The list could go on forever. It is all about possibilities. There are several reasons for listing out all the possible data. Some nurses can't think beyond *"call the doctor."* This takes all responsibility for action and places it on someone else. Nurses are suggesters. We are the ones who say, *"Would you like, have you considered, how about?"* and if they don't know what to suggest, they aren't being as efficient as they should be. Plus, nurses are being held legally responsible for knowing whether or not the doctor wrote the right order, which means that the days of blindly following the doctor's orders are over.

Why you want a piece of data is equally important as *what* you want. When a student requests something, I ask them to tell me why they want it. Why do you want an EKG on this particular patient? Answer: It shows rate, rhythm, infarction, ischemia, extremes of drugs and electrolytes on the myocardium. This keeps the student from reciting the standing orders on a certain type of patient without having any understanding of what the orders mean. It is also important that, if the student can justify the request, it be allowed in. The teacher must have an open mind to creativity when it is within reason. Nothing shuts down critical thinking faster than a teacher who says *"no"* to possibilities because they are not part of the teacher's past experience.

Some of this data is more important than others. How do you decide what is the most important? What signifies oxygenation and perfusion? Physical exam, vital signs, O2 sat, EKG. We could tell the student to do these things and in what order, but there would be no thinking, only rote memorization. Each time, you let the student brainstorm possibilities and then say, "*Now, which are the most important?*" The ones that prove that the patient is oxygenating and perfusing at the same time. All the possibilities need to be in his head so that when the most important are completed, the student has a good idea of what else needs to be done. This is going to vary from patient to patient and rote memorization can't envision all the possibilities. Critical thinking is about possibilities within this context.

Assumption

What assumption have you made about Jack's event? Cardiac? Under reasons for the problem, all possibilities are discussed, but the first to be addressed is the one most likely to kill the patient. Our assumption should be that this is a cardiac event. If the student has chosen any other assumption to act on, the teacher should listen to the student's reasoning for his choice but guide him to the event most likely to kill the patient – and that is always a lethal dysrythmia. Novices do not have the past experience necessary to properly prioritize a patient's problems. You have to help them by telling them that the option they go after first is the one that will kill the patient, then the one that will maim the patient, then those that will harm the patient, and everything else lines up after that.

Other Reasons for the Problem

What else could it possibly be? The assumption is the starting point, but it is important to have other possibilities in mind. As new data comes in, it can change the direction of the treatment. What is missing? When it shows up, it can change everything. Has the radiologist read the X-ray yet? Did we get the old chart? Are the labs back? When these things show up, they can change the direction of care. This is one reason why possibilities as to what is causing this problem to occur are important. If you aren't thinking of other possibilities even as you act on your assumption, you might discount the new information as irrelevant. This is called *early closure* in problem-solving. The mind is made up and no amount of new information will open it back up.

Other things that could be causing Jack's problems include esophageal spasm, gall bladder, reflux disease, MI, aortic dissection, stomach ulcers – and on and on. Could we have done this with the medications we gave the patient? Sure. This section is simply possibilities. Pneumonia? Pneumothorax? Sepsis? Sure, all are possibilities. As data comes in, it will point us to the correct cause.

Patient Goal

What would you like to see as an outcome for the patient? To determine the goal for Jack, we revisit the problem list and see what is keeping him from oxygenating and perfusing at the same time. His current problems are: hr and bp down, rr is up, the patient is cold, clammy, and diaphoretic, Lopressor and NTG on board, and chest pain. Which should we set as the goal?

If we chose relieving the chest pain as the goal, will that necessarily make the heart rate and blood pressure come up and make the cold, clammy, and diaphoretic go away? No. If we get the heart rate and blood pressure up, can we make the cold, clammy, diaphoretic go away? The respiratory rate came down (it is probably a response to tissue hypoxia and the resultant metabolic acidosis), so did the chest pain go away? Yes. The goal should be the event that corrects the most of the problems and gets our patient to oxygenate and perfuse at the same time. Let's get Jack's heart rate and blood pressure up. We now know exactly what we are going to do and the novice has followed a logical progression to get here.

Methods

There are things we can do to help us reach our goal, which in this case is to get the heart rate and blood pressure up. Because you should never do anything to anyone unless you have a very good idea of what can happen, we are going to also list the positive and negative side effects of each of our methods.

Method 1 - **Oxygen**
  Positive effect – O2 saturation comes up
  Negative effect – nothing
  (Wow, the negative here is very benign. I might do this right away)

Method 2 - **Fluids**
  Positive effect – blood pressure comes up
  Negative effect – fluid overload
  The negative here is more caustic; I might want more information before I act

Method 3 - **Atropine**
  Positive effect – Heart rate comes up
  Negative effect – increases myocardial oxygen consumption

Method 4 - **Dopamine**
  Positive effect – Heart rate and blood pressure come up
  Negative effect – greatly increases myocardial oxygen consumption, causing the patient to infarct

Method 5 - **External pacemaker**
  Positive effect – heart rate comes up
  Negative effect – hurts, sedation required, capture difficult in people with deep chests or large breasts

Method 6 - **Internal pacemaker**
  Positive effect – heart rate comes up
  Negative effect – very invasive, many complications, takes time to get the right people there with the right equipment for insertion

Method 7 - **Call a code or call for the rapid response team**
  Positive effect – you get help
  Negative effect – it takes time for them to arrive
  The sooner I call, the quicker they will arrive

Method 8 - **Transfer the patient to the CCU/ICU**
> *Positive effect* – gone to a higher standard of care
> *Negative effect* – dies in route

Method 9 - Send the patient to the cath lab
> *Positive effect* – positive diagnosis and intervention
> *Negative effect* – it takes time to get the team in and the patient dies in the lab

Method 10 - Morphine
> *Positive effect* – chest pain relieved
> *Negative effect* – decrease in blood pressure
> **(This negative effect is very caustic. I will hesitate to do this)**

Look at all the things we can possible do for Jack. There were four things listed that would directly increase his heart rate: atropine, dopamine, internal and external pacemakers. The complications and availability of the treatment make some more desirable than others. Putting oxygen on the patient looks benign; let's do that immediately. Morphine looks like it might make the blood pressure problem worse. Let's hold on that method. If a cardiologist is in the room with an internal pacing catheter in her hand, are you going to ask her to leave the room? What you do depends on what you have available. Do not teach 1, 2, 3. Teach "here is our goal and here are our possibilities." What you do depends on what you have available and the special circumstances surrounding this patient.

When I am doing a patient care scenario for a class, I like to throw in a possibility that they have not considered. With Jack, I asked the class if they would like to know what was wrong with Jack in real life. When they say yes, I told them that Jack had a vasovagal response – a profound drop in the heart rate and blood pressure caused by stimulating the parasympathetic system, in this case by gagging when the NTG was placed under his tongue. Few students will think of this possibility and I would not have thought of it except that I had a patient with this problem. Experience is the teacher. Jack was nauseated – that was it. The vasovagal response was prolonged by the cardiac medications we had given him.

There was nothing wrong with Jack's heart; it was all in his gut. Was the student wrong to make the assumption that it was a cardiac event? No, it is your heart that will kill you and you must eliminate that variable first. Assuming the worst buys time for data to come in.

Alice

Alice is a 66-year-old woman with a history of CAD, HTN, PVD, and is a CO_2 retaining COPDer. She smokes 3 packs of cigarettes a day, and has a very sedentary life style – she loves reality TV shows. Her 34-year-old son, his live-in girlfriend (when she is out of rehab) and their two-year-old twins live with Alice. Last month, Alice was out cutting firewood (she didn't want to wake her son because he had been up late the night before) when she developed chest pain. She sat down, had a couple of cigarettes, and the pain went away.

Alice was admitted to your floor for an ORIF of the left ankle that she fractured when she fell off her porch. It is day three post-op and she is confused, restless, and agitated.

Current problems for Alice: confused, restless, agitated, post-op, fractured bone, CAD, COPD with CO_2 retention, current smoker, HTN, PVD, sedentary life style, family stress. These things we know about Alice from her admit diagnosis and H&P.

Potential problems for Alice: myocardial ischemia, rhythm disturbance, CVA pulmonary embolus, pneumonia, CO_2 narcosis, DVT, decreased healing, skin breakdown, nutritional imbalance, risk for falls and further trauma, aspiration

The worst thing that could happen to Alice is that she would have a lethal dysrythmia and die because she was hypoxic and/or had myocardial ischemia. She also faces other problems with nutrition, skin breakdown, falls and probably other things you can think of.

Data needed: EGK, vital signs, O2 sat, ABG, physical exam including heart and lung sounds, neuro assessment, CXR, CTs to R/O PE and intracranial problems, medication list with narcotic doses and times, allergies, social service work up, alcohol consumption?, what are the circumstances surrounding the fall from her porch?, CBC, lactate level, BUN, Cr, lytes, blood glucose, old chart, etc.

These are things we would like to know about Alice. These are things that will help point us in the right direction for our assumption and potential reasons for the problem. We must prove that Alice is oxygenating and perfusing at the same time, just like we did for Jack in the previous example.

Data needed and reasons for the problem go hand in hand. If you think the patient may be septic, have you asked for anything that would prove or disprove sepsis? Did you get a CBC, lactate level or blood cultures? By the same token, if you asked for a chest x ray, do you think a possibility is pneumonia?

Assumption: This is abnormal behavior for Alice and needs to be evaluated.

That this is abnormal behavior for Alice is crucial for action to take place. "She's been that way since I got here," drives me right up the wall. What is normal for this patient? Bad things happen when the assumption is made that this particular behavior is normal for this patient when it is not.

Reasons for the problem: What else could it possibly be? Everything we can think of causes a change in mentation. We will look at diseases, but don't forget drugs – things we gave her or things she is used to having but hasn't gotten since she came into the hospital. What about sleep deprivation? It is day three post-op, just the right time for sleep problems to crop up. Other possibilities are pneumonia, pulmonary embolus, hypovolemia for whatever reason, CVA, sepsis, electrolyte imbalance, myocardial infarction, reaction to the narcotics, antibiotics, or other medications, change in environment causing disorientation, alcohol withdrawal, etc.

Goal of Therapy: Return Alice to her normal state of being

Methods

Method 1 – **O2**
>   *Positive effect* – oxygen saturation increases
>   *Negative effect* – nothing; with time the CO_2 may go up

Method 2 – **Elevate the head of the bed**
>   *Positive effect* – increase oxygenation
>   *Negative effect* – lower blood pressure, possibly
>   contraindicated if there is an extreme situation like increased
>   intracranial pressure, spinal fracture, etc

Method 3 – **Straighten pt**
>   *Positive effect* – increase oxygenation and perfusion
>   *Negative effect* – none

Method 4 – **Give Narcan**
>   *Positive effect* – remove effect of narcotics
>   *Negative effect* – sudden, severe pain

Method 5 – **Intubate if necessary**
>   *Positive effect* – control airway, increase oxygenation
>   *Negative effect* – invasive, requires respirator, many complications

Method 6 – **BiPAP**
>   *Positive effect* – increases oxygenation
>   *Negative effect* – agitates patient, making hypoxia worse

Method 7 – **Antibiotics if appropriate**
>   *Positive effect* – remove sepsis
>   *Negative effect* – damage liver and kidneys, allergy

Method 8 – **Fluids**
>   *Positive effect* – increase blood pressure
>   *Negative effect* – fluid overload

Method 9 – **Side rails up, sitter**
>   *Positive effect* – keep patient from falling
>   *Negative effect* – agitate patient, patient may still fall

Alice has a very complex problem and there is not too much we can do until some of the data comes in. We will definitely increase her oxygenation by raising the head of the bed and straightening her into an upright position. In her altered mental status, falls are a real problem, so let's get the side rails up and possibly a sitter or a posey belt depending on her level of consciousness. We will not leave this patient until we know what is going on and have reversed its effects. Our blood gas comes back showing hypoxia with a higher than normal CO2 and the chest X-ray shows pneumonia. Alice ends up on BiPAP with antibiotics.

What happened to Alice is what all of our patients are at risk for: inactivity and narcotics post-op added up to bad lungs and poor pulmonary toilet = pneumonia. Alice didn't get up enough, used her PCA too much, had a incentive spirometer sitting at her bedside not being used and had really bad lungs – a recipe for disaster. But it could have been sleep deprivation, DTs, narcotics, or any of the other reasons we listed as possibilities. In the example of Jack everything pointed at this heart, whereas for Alice nothing really pointed anywhere until more data came in. This is why hypothesis generation or possibilities are so important. The student must always be saying, "What else could it be?"

Past experience places expectation on the current situation. As I was describing Alice did you picture her and her family in your mind? Was it flattering? Her son? What did you think of him? And the girlfriend in and out of rehab. My goodness! Two-year-old twins? What must Alice's home life have been like? And how did Alice come to fall off the porch? In a drunken confrontation with her son?

Let me tell you about Alice. Alice is a pillar of her community and very active in her church. She is the secretary-treasurer of the local Habitat for Humanity. Alice has one flaw; when she was a teenager, she started smoking and has never been able to stop. Why was her son up late that night and she didn't want to wake him? He had been working on a Habitat house late into the night to get it finished, so the new owner could move in and get her children into school the next day. What kind of rehab was the girlfriend in – physical rehab. She was injured working on a Habitat house. How did Alice come to break her ankle in the first place? One of the twins (adopted from Ethiopia) had crawled up onto the porch railing in a precarious position. Alice ran to get the child, tripped on the knitting she was doing for the Salvation Army, fell off the porch and broke her ankle.

Now, why would you have thought of Alice and her family the way you did? Because of your past experience, but see how it places expectation on current situation? If the diagnosis is cirrhosis of the liver or HIV, what kind of patient do you see? Patients face tremendous prejudice from us because we think we know who they are based on an H&P or diagnosis. Be careful.

This Model for Critical Thinking would have you believe that problem solving is linear, but there is nothing linear about critical thinking. Rather than being linear, it is a series of loops winding back on themselves as data comes in and has to be responded to. We have a power PICC into a patient and his CVP is very high. We had thought he was hypovolemic when he really was overloaded. We stopped the fluid bolus and gave him some Lasix.

The problem is that you cannot teach novices with a series of loops doubling back on themselves. You have to pull things apart so they can see and understand them. As they progress through the stages of proficiency, they will begin to understand complexities and context, but not at the beginning. It can be very difficult for the experienced nurse to pull the complex loops apart so the novice can see them. The Critical Thinking Model is an aid for both groups to help each other learn. Data has proven that the model increases critical thinking in those who need it most – those with the lowest critical thinking abilities. If you give novices a way to organize their thought processes, they will increase their critical thinking abilities.

The model needs to be started early and used often. Introducing it at the beginning of class but then never or, at best, infrequently using it is not conducive to building critical thinking skills. Introducing the model at the end of the learning experience will also not help the student's critical thinking abilities. It must be used often enough by a teacher who sees possibilities in order to be effective. Early on, it will be a paper and pen exercise, but eventually it will become ingrained in the student's thought process. Then it will become verbal and eventually will become internalized. At this point, you have taught critical thinking skills to your student – every teacher's dream.

Summary

Subclinical signs precede clinical signs. If I had to choose only one vital sign to follow, it wouldn't be blood pressure – it would be heart rate, because the heart rate is a direct look into the patient's heart at stroke volume. Heart rate goes up and down in response to volume (preload), contractility, metabolic demand, and workload (afterload). Increasing heart rate is the first indicator that patients may be fluid overloaded, hypovolemic, infected, and/ or hypoxic.

Because the heart and lungs are so closely tied together, when the heart rate begins to climb, the respiratory rate begins to climb also. Respiratory rate starting to climb is the first sign of respiratory distress, and is also the first sign of patients going into congestive heart failure, ARDS, or other hypoxic events. All of this happens due to the body doing its best to compensate for the lactic acidosis being produced on a cellular level. Septic patients will show this early sign. And beware of drugs that mask the sympathetic response like calcium channel and beta blockers, because if they're onboard, you won't see the heart rate or blood pressure respond as they would without them.

How long the subclinical signs last will vary from patient to patient. The younger and healthier they are when they enter their events, the longer they will be able to compensate. Some patients seem to crash and burn all at once, but if you go back and look at their vital signs, subclinical indications have often been present for hours. Good compensatory mechanisms will allow patients to hide overt symptoms from you. But the signs are there if you know what to look for – heart rate and respiratory rate starts to climb, and for the patient going into CHF, urine output becomes less than it was before.

Our patients are sicker than ever, and there are fewer and fewer nurses involved in direct patient care. The nurse must look for trends in vital signs to see catastrophe coming. Do not rely on your nurse's aide to report abnormal vital signs. They are trained to take vital signs, not to interpret them. It is the nurse who frequently stands between the patient and an emergency

Having knowledge is great, but the nurse must care enough to act on the patient's behalf. Critical thinking allows the nurse to look at the event by considering a series of possibilities, not just the most likely ones. Context is crucial, and also must be considered. Look for the signs of compensation in the body – these are the subclinical signs of impending doom. Then act to prevent the crisis. It is not the nurse's job to run a good code; it is the nurse's job to prevent the code from ever happening.

References

American College of Cardiology Foundation, American Heart Association. (2009). Practice Guidelines for the Diagnosis and Management of Heart Failure in Adults. Retrieved June 1, 2011 from http://circ ahajournals.org/cgi/reprint,CIRCULATIONAHA.109.192064

Benner, P. (1984, 2001) From Novice to Expert. Upper Saddle River, NJ: Prentice Hall.

Benner, P. and Tanner, C. (1987) Clinical Judgement: How Expert Nurses Use Intuition. *American Journal of Nursing*, January, 23-31.

Brookfield, S. (1987). Developing Critical Thinkers. Open University Press: Milton Keynes.

Dolan, J. (1996) Critical Care Nursing: Clinical Management Through the Nursing Process, Philadelphia, PA: F.A. Davis Co.

Dossey, B. (2000). Florence Nightingale: Mystic, Visionary, Healer. Philadelphia, PA: Lippincott, Williams and Wilkins.

Falcione, P. (1990). Critical Thinking: A Statement of Expert Consensus for the Purposes of Educational and Instruction. Millbrae, CA: The California Academic Press.

Gladwell, M. (2007). Blink:The Power of Thinking Without Thinking. New York, NY: Back Bay Books.

Gender related differences in cardiac response to supine exercise assessed by radionuclide angiography, *American Journal of Cardiology* 13(3), 624-9 on March 1, 1989.

Goleman, G. (1995-2006). Emotional Intelligence. New York, NY: Bantam.

Gosling, J., et al (2002). Human Anatomy: Color Atlas and Text. 4th Ed. St. Louis, MO: Mosby.

Guyton, A; Hall, W. (2011). Textbook of Medical Physiology. 12th Ed. St. Louis, MO: Mosby.

Hancock, J. (2010) Cell Signalling. New York, NY: Oxford University Press.

Kapit, W. (1987). The Physiology Coloring Book. Cambridge, MA: Harper Collins Publishers.

Kumar, V. (2009) Robbins and Cotran: Pathologic Basis of Disease. Philadelphia, PA: W.B. Saunders Company

Lewis,S. (2003). Medical-Surgical Nursing: Assessment and Management of Clinical Problems. St. Louis, MO: Mosby.

McCance, K.; Hueter, S. (2005). Pathophysiology: The Biological Basis for Disease in Adults and Children. 5th Ed. St. Louis, MO: Mosby.

References

McNeill, J. and Turlock, A.(1855). Report of the Inquiry into the Supplies of the British Army in the Crimea. Retrieved June 1, 2011 from www.crimeantexts.org.uk/sources/reports/mnt00000.html

Mikati, I. (2010) Heart Disease in Women. Retrieved June 1, 2011 from www.nlm.nih.gov/medlineplus/ency/article/007188.htm

National Coalition for Women with Heart Disease. Retrieved June 1, 2011 from www.womenheart.org. Data from the National Center for Health Statistics; National Heart, Lung, and Blood Institute, and the American Heart Association.

Nightingale, F. (1859-1992). Notes on Nursing. Philadelphia, PA: JB Lippincott.

Paula, R. (2009). Emergent Management of Acute Compartment Syndrome. Retrieved June 1, 2011 from www.emedicine.medscape.com/article/307668.

Porth, C. (2008). Pathophysiology: Concepts of Altered Health States. Philadelphia, PA: J.B. Lippincott Company.

Rensberger, B. (1996) Life Itself: Exploring the Realm of the Living Cell. New York, NY, Oxford University Press.

Russel. W. (1856). The War. London: G. Routledge and Co.

Scheffer, B.; Rubenfield, M. (2000). A Consensus Statement on Critical Thinking in Nursing. Journal of Nursing Education, No; 39(8) 352-9.

Sousa, D. (2008) How the Brain Learns. Thousand Oaks, CA: Corwin Press.

Tanner, C. (2006). Thinking like a Nurse: A Research Based Model of Clinical Judgment in Nursing. *Journal of Nursing Education.* 45(6), 204-11.

Watson, G. and Glaser, E. (1980). Watson-Glaser Critical thinking Aprasial. San Antonio, TX: The Psychological Corporation.

Whiteside, C. (1997). A Model for Teaching Critical Thinking in the Clinical Setting. *Dimensions of Critical Care Nursing.* 16(3) 152-62.

Yamada, A, et al (2007). Gender Differences in Ventricular Volumes and Left Ventricular Ejection Fraction Estimated by Myocardial Perfusion Imaging. Retrieved June 1, 2011 from www.scielo.br/pdf/abc/v88n3/en_a06v88n.

About the Author

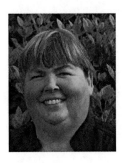

Carol Whiteside, *MSN, PhD*

Carol Whiteside has been a nurse since 1972. She is a Clinical Nurse Specialist, a Cardiovascular Nurse Specialist and recieved her PhD in Educational Leadership with her dissertation titled *The Leadership of Florence Nightingale as Depected in Her Letters from the Crimean War.* Carol has been a staff nurse, cath lab manager, nursing supervisor and director of education. She previously worked in trauma, burn, pediatriac, neonatal, medical/surgical, and cardiac ICUs.

Carol has also been a preceptor and a clinical nursing instructor. Additionally, she is a nurse entrepreneur presenting courses in critical thinking and a variety of nursing topics. Carol has the unique ability to combine her vast clinical background and information with critical thinking strategies and has been a sought-after international speaker for many years.